Jun Takada
Nuclear Hazards in the World

Jun Takada

Nuclear Hazards in the World

Field Studies on Affected Populations
and Environments

With 89 Figures and 28 Tables

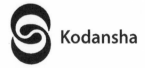 Kodansha   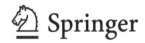 Springer

Professor Jun Takada
Sapporo Medical University
School of Medicine
Minami 1 Jou, Nishi 17 Chome
Sapporo 060-8556
Japan

ISBN 4-06-211076-8 Kodansha Ltd., Tokyo

ISBN-10   3-540-25272-X Springer Berlin Heidelberg New York
ISBN-13   978-3-540-25272-6 Springer Berlin Heidelberg New York

Cover picture: Nuclear explosion in Hiroshima, August 6, 1945.
© Research Institute for Radiation Biology and Medicine, Hiroshima University,
Library of Hiroshima University, 2004

Library of Congress Control Number: 2005921902

Springer is a part of Springer Science + Business Media.

springeronline.com

© Kodansha Ltd. and Springer-Verlag Berlin Heidelberg 2005
Printed in Japan

Cover design: Erich Kirchner, Heidelberg, Germany

Printed on acid-free paper   SPIN: 10843361   30/3141/di - 5 4 3 2 1 0

Acknowledgments

The fieldwork has been collaborated not only by scientists but also by ordinary
people in the world.
The scientific work was supported by several organizations.

Japan
Masanobu Sakanoue (deceased)   LLRL, Kanazawa University, Tatsunokuchi
Masaharu Hoshi   RIRBM Hiroshima University, Hiroshima
Tuneto Nagatomo   Nara Education University, Nara
Masayoshi Yamamoto   LLRL, Kanazawa University, Tatsunokuchi
Tetsuji Imanaka   KRL Kyoto University, Kumatori
Kazuhisa Komura   LLRL, Kanazawa University, Tatsunokuchi
Nanao Kamada   RIRBM Hiroshima University, Hiroshima
Toshiaki Mitsugashira   Tohoku University, Oarai
Shunichi Yamashita   Nagasaki University, Nagasaki
Kunihiko Shinohara   Japan Nuclear Cycle Development, Tokaimura
Yoshitsugu Morishita   Japan Nuclear Cycle Development, Tsuruga
Yasuhide Sakakibara   Japan Nuclear Cycle Development, Tsuruga
Hiroshi Hiroi   Japan Nuclear Cycle Development, Tsuruga
Hironobu Gotoh   The Chugoku Electric Power Co. Inc.
Kousei Shimada   BunBun Project, Hayama
Taniko Shimizu   BunBun Project, Hayama
Shigeyuki Watanabe   BunBun Project, Tokyo
Hiroko Maki   Sasagawa Memorial Health Foundation, Tokyo

Russia
V.F. Stepanenko   Medical Radiological Research Center of
                                RAMS, Obninsk
A.E. Kondrashov   Medical Radiological Research Center of
                                RAMS, Obninsk

D.V. Petin	Medical Radiological Research Center of RAMS, Obninsk
V. Skvortsov	Medical Radiological Research Center of RAMS, Obninsk
A. Ivanikov	Medical Radiological Research Center of RAMS, Obninsk
V.P. Snykov (deceased)	SPA TYPHOON, Obninsk
Yu. Konstantinov	Institute of Radiation Hygiene, St. Petersburg
P.V. Ramzaev	Institute of Radiation Hygiene, St. Petersburg
Yu.I. Gavrilin	Institute of Biophysics, Moscow
V. Sharov	Urals Medical Academy Additional Education, Urals
M. Degteva	Urals Radiation Center for Radiation Medicine, Urals
N.G. Bougrov	Urals Radiation Center for Radiation Medicine, Urals
V.E. Stepanov	Yakut State University, Yakut
D.P. Yefremov	The Ministry of Nature Protection, Yakut

Belarus
| V.E. Shevchuk | Gomel Branch of Institute of Radiation Medicine, Gomel |
| Yu. V. Sushko | Radiation Research Station, Masani |

Kazakhstan
B.I. Gusev	Kazakh Scientific Research Institute for Radiation Medicine and Ecology, Semipalatinsk
A.K. Sekerbaev	Kazakh Scientific Research Institute for Radiation Medicine and Ecology, Semipalatinsk
R. Rosenson	Kazakh Scientific Research Institute for Radiation Medicine and Ecology, Semipalatinsk
K. Apsarikov	Kazakh Scientific Research Institute for Radiation Medicine and Ecology, Semipalatinsk
N.J. Tchaijunusova	Kazakh Scientific Research Institute for Radiation Medicine and Ecology, Semipalatinsk
Z. Zhumadilov	Semipalatinsk Medical Academy, Semipalatinsk
K. Zhumadilov	National Nuclear Center, Kurchatov

Marshall Islands
E. Ned	Boat Limanman (North Star), Mejatto Island
N. Anjain	The former Mayer of Rongelap Island, Mejatto Island
N. Bigler (deceased)	Pacific International Inc., Rongelap Island

Financial Support
Ministry of Education, Science, Sports and Cultures Japan
The Nippon Foundation
Hiroshima International Council for Medical Care of the Radiation-exposed

The author should be appreciate his wife Midori and his parents Seiji and Hisako for their lot of support. He is also grateful Kazuo Koeda (deceased), Kazuya Yanagida and Ippei Ohta for giving an opportunity of publication from Kodansha.

Preface

Science and technology have made great progress in energy, information communication and life in the 20th century. Recognition of the negative aspects and the serious efforts to minimize their influence on society is important in the 21st century.

Since the beginning of the last century, nuclear science and technology have been developed by advanced countries such as the United States of America, the former USSR, UK, France and Japan. This has had great impact on the world, providing the ultimate weapon to human beings, a new kind of energy, as well as new medical and industrial technologies.

Nuclear science and technology were first applied to the generation of electricity on a commercial scale in USSR in 1954 and spread throughout the world. More than 400 nuclear power plants are operating worldwide at the beginning of the 21st century. If the fast-breeder reactor is successfully put to safe practical use, it will alleviate the energy problem for many years.

On the other hand, many people are concerned about the occurrence of nuclear disasters and radiation exposure. Historically, the use of nuclear technology has produced several severe disasters resulting in long-term pollution in the world, such as combat use in Hiroshima and Nagasaki, a large number of weapons test explosions and the Chernobyl reactor accident.

Although we have been informed of the social impact by the media, the negative aspects, including effects on health, environments, agriculture, etc. are not scientifically clear so far. The reason is the small amount of research work conducted compared with that on the positive applications, and complicated phenomena involving biological and environmental components with many unknown factors. Moreover, many cases of nuclear disasters were military and veiled in secrecy.

This book provides a general overview of nuclear disasters, updated individual and summarized information on several major nuclear hazards in the world to a wide audience. The study of nuclear hazards based on field work was carried out by a single scientist using common measurement methods between 1995 and 2002.

The sites include hazardous areas such the Techa River area polluted by the plutonium production complex Mayak around the Semipalatinsk nuclear weapon test site, Rongelap Island contaminated by fallout from a Bravo 15Mt thermonuclear test in Bikini, underground nuclear explosions for industrial application conducted in Siberia, the restricted control zone after the Chernobyl accident, Tokaimura exposed by a criticality accident and Hiroshima. Moreover, a simulation of nuclear weapon terrorism in the city is discussed in the Appendix. The readers can study facts regarding the initial stages of a disaster, radiation exposure of the public and interventions for radiation protection. The author also discusses some remarkable characteristics of hazards which occurred after a nuclear disaster. This monograph provides a realistic evaluation of radiation exposures of nuclear hazards throughout the world and an insight into aspects of recovery from such hazards.

This volume is recommended for graduate students as well as specialists in both private and public sectors working in environmental science and technology, food and agricultural sciences and technology, medical science, radiation hygiene, radiation protection and nuclear science and technology.

Jun Takada
Sapporo 2005

Contents

1

Overview of Nuclear Disasters

Over 2,400 nuclear explosions were conducted worldwide during the cold war between the USA and USSR since July 1945. The total yield of 530 Mt was 35,000 times that of the Hiroshima atomic bomb. Surface and underground nuclear explosions caused radioactive pollution locally in ground and water systems. Fission products and plutonium with long half-lives are nuclear hazards for local populations. However, the radiological situation is still unclear in many areas that suffered nuclear disaster. There was also nuclear waste pollution from plutonium production facilities for weapons development. Release of radioactivity twenty times that of the Hiroshima bomb was reported in the Chernobyl accident of the former USSR. Other nuclear disasters have also occurred at various nuclear facilities. Over 400 nuclear power plants are in operation throughout the world at

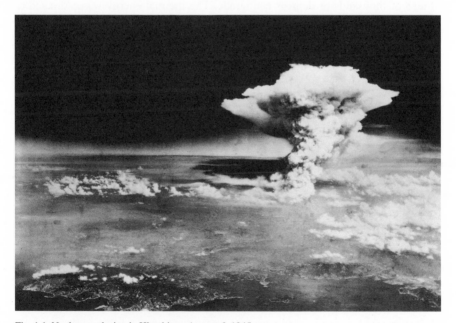

Fig. 1.1 Nuclear explosion in Hiroshima, August 6, 1945.
[©Research Institute for Radiation Biology and Medicine, Hiroshima University, Library of Hiroshima University, 2004]

present. This application is a peaceful one, but several accidents have happened. In this chapter, we first review the Hiroshima nuclear weapon and the physical phenomena of nuclear explosions. This is followed by a brief summary of accidents at nuclear facilities which are relevant for many countries seeking the peaceful application of nuclear power.

1.1 The Tragedy in Hiroshima

Hiroshima and Nagasaki were attacked by nuclear bombs exploded at an altitude of about 500 m. A two-kilometer zone in both cities was destroyed by shock wave and thermal radiation.[1] Ground zero near the hypocenter was irradiated by high energy gamma rays and neutrons.

Uranium-235 (U-235) was used in the Hiroshima nuclear weapon with an output of an equivalent of TNT 15 kt.[2] This exploded in the sky 580 m above the surface. A 2-km radius of the city was destroyed by shock wave and thermal radiation. Gamma rays and neutrons of high energy resulting from the nuclear fission chain reaction caused radiation exposure of the population at ground zero.

Air expansion by super high pressure of hundreds of thousands of atoms at the epicenter[*1] caused the explosion. The wind speed was estimated to be 280 m/s at ground zero.[3] The edge of the blast moves in a shock wave. After 30 seconds, it reached a distance of 11 km from the hypocenter.[*2] Later, when the blast moving outward stopped, a weak blast flowing inward formed a mushroom cloud.

The fireball formed by the nuclear fission chain reaction reached a maximum of tens of thousands of degrees centigrade. The thermal energy was estimated to be 100 cal/m² at ground zero and 1.8 cal/m² at a distance of 3.5 km from the

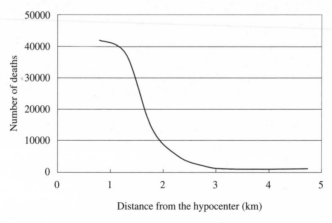

Fig. 1.2 The number deaths within 0.5 km as a function of distance from the hypocenter.[3]

---

*1 The center of a burst of a nuclear weapon.
*2 The point on the surface of land vertically below or above the center of a burst of a nuclear weapon. This term sometimes used for ground zero.

hypocenter.[3] The thermal wounds from exposed skin affected the population within a distance of 3.5 km. Those within a 1.2 km radius who were not sheltered suffered fatal heat injuries.

In the case of the Hiroshima nuclear weapon, residents within a 2-km radius received a remarkably high dose by the initial radiation from this aerial nuclear explosion. Radioactivity was also induced on the ground surface by the absorption of neutrons from the epicenter. This induction of radioactivity decreased rapidly. The dose rate at ground zero due to induction radioactivity was estimated to be about 10 mSv/h one day after the explosion, 0.01 mSv/h after one week and about 0.1 μSv/h after one year.[4]

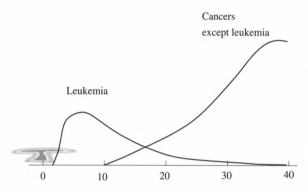

Fig. 1.3 Cancers of survivors after the bombing in Hiroshima.
[Reproduced with permission from Hiroshima International Council for Health Care of the Radiation Exposed, *Effects of A-Bomb Radiation on the Human Body*, Bunkodo Co., Ltd.-Harwood Academic Publishers (1992)]

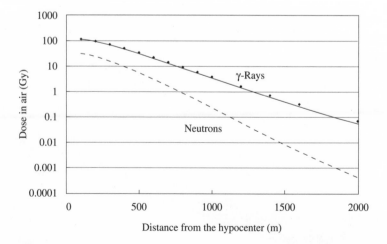

Fig. 1.4 DS86.
[Reproduced with permission from M.L. Gritzner, W.A. Woolson, *US-Japan Joint Reassessment of Atomic Bomb Radiation Dosimetry in Hiroshima and Nagasaki, Final Report*, Vol.2, p.342, Hiroshima Radiation Effects Research Foundation (1987)]

In Hiroshima, 140,000 people died by December of 1945. As for the health effects of radiation exposure, there were not only acute radiation effects but late effects as well.

Radiation dose was evaluated as a function of distance. In 1965, the dose was estimated (T65D) but it was reevaluated by a Japan-U.S. joint project in 1986 (DS86).[2] According to DS86, the approximate dose on the skin surface at a distance of 1,000 meters was 4 Gy from gamma rays and 0.2 Gy from neutrons. Gamma rays reach distant places. Because neutrons lose energy by collision with hydrogen atoms in air of approximately the same mass, they are not a large component of radiation exposure at large distances.

1.2 Survivors

There were survivors within 500 meters from the hypocenter in Hiroshima. Seventy-eight survivors (48 men, 30 women) were confirmed in the area by an investigation conducted in 1968-1970. Their age composition on the day of the bombing was three who were less than nine years old, twenty-four 10–19 year-olds, fifteen 20–29 year-olds, sixteen 30–39 year-olds, seventeen 40–49 year-olds, and three 50–59 year-olds. These survivors were in concrete buildings, in a vault and in a streetcar. That there were seven survivors in a train is remarkable.

Research on these survivors was implemented from 1972 by a project, "General Medical Research on Survivors within Close Range of the Bombing," of the Research Institute of Radiation Biology and Medicine of Hiroshima University.[5] The average dose of these survivors was evaluated to be 2.8 Gy from

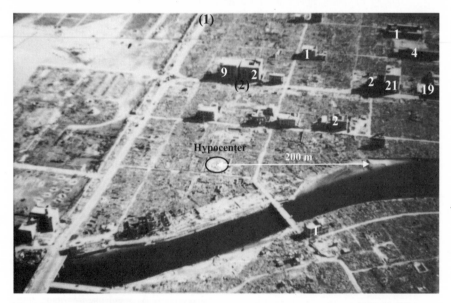

Fig. 1.5 The number of survivors at ground zero.
[©Research Institute for Radiation Biology and Medicine, Hiroshima University, Library of Hiroshima University, 2004]

the research on aberrations of chromosomes conducted by Dr. N. Kamada. Dose outdoors without any radiation shield is estimated to be more than 30 Gy. This means that survivors were fairly well shielded from radiation by the walls of buildings and other barriers. Most of them suffered acute radiation syndrome.

In the 25 years between 1972 and 1997, number of deaths was 45. The age distribution of those who died is as follows: four were less than 60 years old, 10 were in their 60s, 15 in their 70s, 13 in their 80s and three in their 90s. The

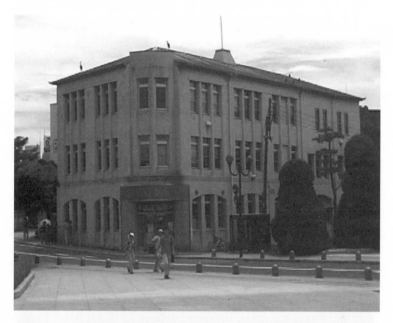

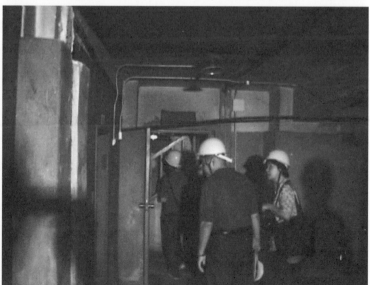

Fig. 1.6 Rest house and the basement (170 m from the hypocenter) that protected a survivor.

average age of death is 74.4 years old. This indicates no remarkable shortening of life span.

Eizo Nomura, a staff member of the Hiroshima Prefecture Fuel Distribution Regulation Association, which was 170 m from the hypocenter, was one of the survivors. At the time of the bombing, he entered a clerical room in the basement to obtain a document. Nomura escaped from the vault in the darkness and ran from ground zero where water from the Otagawa River reached high up to the sky. Nomura lived to be 84 years old until his death in 1982. The concrete which surrounded the vault and thick earth prevented the shock wave, thermal radiation, and ionizing radiation from affecting him. This building, which is on the edge of Motoyasu Bridge near the Atomic Bomb Dome, is now used as a rest house in Hiroshima Peace Park. The vault is open to visitors.

1.3 Physical Phenomena of Nuclear Explosion

Nuclear explosion phenomena are summarized here to better understand the radiation exposure of victims of nuclear explosions. There are two types of nuclear weapons devices: the nuclear fission type and the fusion type.

The fission type instantly induces nuclear fission of uranium (U) or plutonium (Pu) causing a chain reaction to release energy. The nuclides which become the fuel in these elements are uranium (U-235) and plutonium (Pu-239). These are called nuclear fission materials. Air shock, thermal radiation and nuclear radiation comprise about 50%, 35% and 15% respectively, of the total released energy from the nuclear explosion in air.[6]

About 15% of the total energy is released as nuclear radiation. Approximately 5% of this constitutes the initial radiation, defined as that produced within one minute of the explosion. The material produced at this time is radioactive and it is called the fission product. The residual nuclear radiation which is emitted over a period of time makes up about 10%. This is mainly due to the fission products. The nuclear fission of uranium and plutonium emits gamma rays and neutrons of high energy.

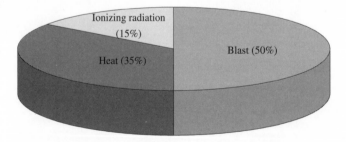

Fig. 1.7 Distribution of energy in a nuclear explosion in air.

The "yield" of a nuclear weapon is the amount of explosive energy the weapon can produce. The usual practice is to state the yield in terms of the quantity of TNT that generates the same amount of energy when it explodes. The energy yield of the complete fission of nuclear fission material of 56 g produces the same amount of explosive energy as 1 kt of TNT.[6] Thus, a 20-kt nuclear weapon is one which produces the same amount of energy as an explosion of 20 kt of TNT. The Hiroshima atomic bomb which the U.S. used in 1945 was the equivalent of 15 kt of TNT. The quantity of U-235 that completed fission was only about 800 grams.

High temperature gas which consists of radioactive material and weapon material rises to the sky as it expands. The fireball gradually cools and becomes shaped like a cloud. Ninety percent radioactivity is included in the mushroom umbrella. Radioactivity in the ground was induced by the capture of neutrons and radiated from the epicenter. At the same time, the surface of the earth was burned by thermal radiation and fires occurred in the city. Thus radioactive materials at ground zero were carried toward the sky by the updraft. This formed the trunk of the nuclear mushroom cloud. Ten percent radioactivity was included in this part.

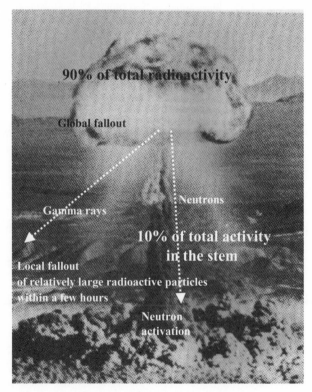

Fig. 1.8 Radioactivity and radiation from the nuclear explosion.
[Photo : ©UP San]

Nuclear fusion reactions can be brought on by very high temperatures. This is called the "thermonuclear process." For example, two deuterium nuclei combine to form the nucleus of a heavier element, helium, with the release of energy. The fusion of all the nuclei in 17 g of deuterium releases the same amount of explosive energy as 1 kt of TNT.[6]

In the fusion of nuclei of hydrogen isotopes, neutrons of high energy are emitted. These neutrons can cause fission in plutonium-239 (Pu-239) and are captured in the most abundant isotope (U-238 to produce Pu-239). It is possible to make use of thermonuclear neutrons by surrounding the fusion weapon with a blanket of ordinary uranium. Consequently, association of the appropriate fusion reactions with natural uranium can result in extensive utilization of the latter for the release of energy. A device in which the fission and fusion reactions are combined has been developed. This type of weapon typically releases equal amounts of explosive energy from fission and from fusion. Therefore, this type of weapon also produces a huge amount of fission products.

1.4 The Fireball and Radioactive Cloud

The fission of uranium (or plutonium) and the fusion of isotopes of hydrogen in a nuclear weapon emit a large amount of energy in a very short period of time. Thus the fission products, bomb casting, and other weapon parts are raised to extremely high temperatures, similar to those in the center of the sun. As a result, all the materials are converted into the gaseous state to form a fireball of high temperature and high pressure.

The size of the fireball increases with the energy yield (W) of the nuclear weapon. The fireball radius R for air burst is empirically related to the yield by

$$R = 34 \ W \ (\text{kt})^{0.4} \tag{1.1}$$

per meter unit.[6] If the height of burst is smaller than R, local fallout ceases to be a serious problem. The relation between R and W is plotted in Fig. 1.9. A 15-kt nuclear weapon will have a radius of 99 m. The fireball of the Hiroshima nuclear weapon of 15 kt which exploded at a height of 580 m did not come in contact with the ground. Thus there was no serious local fallout of fission products at ground zero.

The fireball rises to the sky as it expands. It gradually cools and becomes shaped like a cloud. The neutrons emitted from the fireball will irradiate the surface of the city below and induce radioactivity at ground zero.

Depending on the height of the burst and the nature of the terrain below, a strong updraft of inflowing winds, called the "afterwind," is produced in the vicinity of ground zero. Such afterwinds can cause varying amounts of dirt and debris to be sucked up from the surface of the city. At first the rising mass of weapon residues carries the particles upward, but after a time, they begin to fall slowly under the influence of gravity, at rates dependent upon their size.

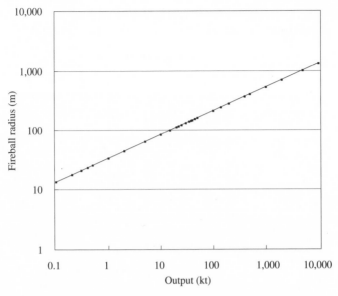

Fig. 1.9 Fireball radius as a function of the energy yield of a nuclear weapon.

1.5 Nuclear Test Explosions

After World War II explosions of nuclear weapons have been implemented 2,419 times with a total TNT equivalent of 530 megatons as of 1998: 1127 times by the U.S., 969 times by the USSR, 57 times by the United Kingdom, 210 times by France, 44 times by China, six times by India, and six times by Pakistan. The development of nuclear weapons continues to this day.

There are many unclear points regarding environmental pollution and inhabitants of surrounding areas exposed to radiation by nuclear weapons tests due to strict information control, depending on the country carrying out the tests. The Science Committee on Problems of the Environment (SCOPE), which is a non-government organization, began the RADTEST project to examine the transport, deposition and human health effects of radioactive fallout from nuclear weapons tests through international, collaborative study in 1993 and published a report, "Nuclear Test Explosion," in 2000.[7]

The main test sites of nuclear weapons were Nevada, Enowetok and Bikini in the Marshall Islands, Pacific, South Atlantic, Alamogordo, Christmas Island area, Johnston Island area (USA), Semipalatinsk (Kazakhstan), the Arctic Circle and Novaya Zemlya (USSR), Emu, Monte Bello Islands, Maralinga, Christmas Island, Malden Island (UK), Reggane, Mururoa, Fangataufa (France), Lob Noll (China), India, Pakistan. The whole earth was polluted by the artificial radioactive material which was released from these nuclear explosions into the atmosphere. The pollution in the northern hemisphere is higher than in the southern hemisphere. The accumulated quantity of the strontium 90 which fell within the range of 30–50 degrees latitude north is from about 2 to 3 kBq/m^2, according to a report of the United Nations Science Committee.[8)]

Table 1.1 Nuclear weapon tests in the world

Country	Nuclear weapon tests			Yield (Mt)		
	Atomospheric	Underground	Total	Atomospheric	Underground	Total
USA	217*	910	1127	154	46	200
USSR	219	750	969	247	38	285
UK	33	24	57	8	2	10
France	50	160	210	10	3	13
China	22	22	44	21	1	22
India		6	6			
Pakistan		6	6			
All countries	541	1878	2419	440	90	530

*Includes two combat uses.

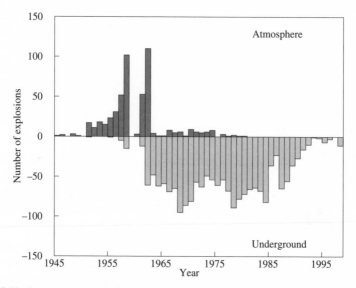

Fig. 1.10 Nuclear weapon test as a function of year throughout the world. Underground tests indicated below the line.
[Reproduced with permission from SCOPE59, *Nuclear Test Explosions*, John Wiley & Sons (2000)]

Nuclear tests are conducted in an unpopulated controlled experimental zone. Therefore, no direct radiation should reach a given radius from the epicenter. However, a huge amount of radioactive material produced by a nuclear explosion may pollute surrounding areas and expose residents to radiation.

1.6 Classification of Nuclear Explosions

Nuclear explosion experiments are classified as ground (surface), air or basement by explosion site. Early nuclear tests were ground explosions by a device placed in a steel tower. A fireball covers the surface raising fine particles of soil polluted by radioactive material into the air. This is the most dangerous type of experiment because a highly radioactive cloud exposes the downwind area to radiation. In the case of aerial explosion by dropping from a war plane, most of the nuclear fission material becomes hot gas that rises into the atmosphere and becomes a source of global nuclear pollution. Neutrons radiating from the hypocenter causes radioactivity at ground zero below. The radioactivity which occurs in this manner forms the trunk of the nuclear mushroom cloud in the hot updraft. Because comparatively large particles are contained in this part, this cloud descends little by a little while moving downwind.

An explosion with a fireball deep under the surface of the earth is classified as an underground nuclear explosion. Such explosions are comparatively safe because plutonium and nuclear fission products are confined underground. Actually, most such explosions occur in wells or caves in mountains. If the explosion occurs in a shallow area, the fireball appears on the surface and in essence becomes a surface explosion. Such a nuclear explosion has occurred historically. Moreover, because the radioactive rare gas which was generated escaped from the surface of the earth, the radiation around the nuclear test site reached a high level for a time.

People are not permitted to reside inside the controlled test areas. For example, the former Soviet Union made the Semipalatinsk Nuclear Test Site within an area of 18,500 km^2, evacuating all residents and livestock. There was no radiation exposure to the population caused by the initial radiation from the

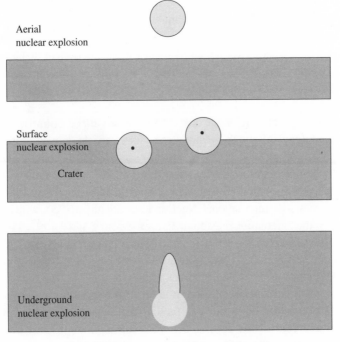

Fig. 1.11 Various types of nuclear explosion tests.

fireball because the radiation did not reach the distant residential areas.

However, there has been enormous radiation exposure to people in distant surrounding areas caused by radioactive clouds containing fission products. Indeed, radiation exposure by the radioactive fallout which occurred from the U.S. 15-Mt thermonuclear explosion on Bikini Atoll in 1954 is especially well known in Japan because a Japanese tuna fishing boat, the *Fukuryuumaru No.5* (*Fortune Dragon No.5*), 150 km from the epicenter, was covered by radioactive material of white powder like snow. This was a mixture of the fine powder of the radiated coral atoll crushed by explosion, nuclear fission products and plutonium. This exposed 23 crew members of the boat to radiation. Also, there was radiation exposure of the population on Rongelap Atoll caused by the fallout. Immediately after the explosion, victims suffered acute radiation effects such as dermatitis, the heaves and diarrhea. On March 3, two days after the explosion, the islanders were rescued by the U.S. Army. This case showed that a surface explosion could cause severe exposure to a population located over 100 km from the center of the explosion.

1.7. Nuclear Facility Accidents and Radiation Exposure

More than 400 nuclear power plants are operating at present throughout the world. The top five producers of nuclear energy are the U.S., France, Japan, Germany and Russia, in this order. For example, the percentage of electricity generated by nuclear power is 77% in France, 57% in Belgium, 44% in Ukraine, 36% in South Korea, 33% in Japan, demonstrating the important role of nuclear power plants. The nuclear power plant employs technology to control nuclear fission chain reaction in a stable manner. The establishment of a safe system is required for peaceful use of nuclear power including processing of fuel, spent fuel and disposal of nuclear waste. One of the greatest challenges of the 21st century is to establish a general safety control system for nuclear energy, including nuclear fuel recycling.

There have been nuclear accidents in the advanced countries involving nuclear technology. Although the number is not large, the impact on society was great. For example, in the Tokaimura criticality accident in Japan in 1999, the sum of damage due to rumors was reported to be U.S. 100 million dollars. However, what was the actual situation? We must examine this disaster scientifically.

There exists the International Nuclear Event Scale (INES), which has been managed by the International Atomic Energy Agency since 1992. Presently 60 countries are members. According to INES, an extraordinary nuclear event is classified into seven levels. The higher levels from 7 to 4 are called accidents. An event lower than level 3 is called an extraordinary event.

In a major accident of maximum level 7, a huge amount of radioactive material is released from a nuclear facility to the outside environment. The Chernobyl accident of the former U.S.S.R. corresponds to this. In the INES classification, the accident of lowest level 4 is an accident without significant off-

Table 1.2 The international nuclear event scale and dose on public

Level	Description	Criteria	Public dose level*	Cases
7	Major accident	A huge amount of radioactive materials released I-131 equivalent of more than several 10 PBq	C	Chernobyl Nuclear Power Plant Accident (The former USSR, Ukraine, 1986)
6	Serious accident	Considerable amount of radioactive materials released I-131 equivalent of several-several tens of PBq		Kyshtym Waste Facility Accident (Russia, 1957)
5	Accident with off-site risk	A limited amount of radioactive materials released I-131 equivalent of several sub-several PBq		Three Mile Island Nuclear Power Plant Accident (USA, 1976)
4	Accident without significant off-site risk	A small amount of radioactive materials released, individual dose of several mSv to public	D	Tokaimura Criticality Accident (Japan, 1999)
3	Serious incident	A very small amount of radioactive materials released, individual dose of several sub mSv to public	E	
2	Incident	No risk to public	F	
1	Anomaly	No risk to public	F	

Levels 7-4: Accidents Levels 3 and 2: Incidents Level 1: Anomalies
* This dose level was added by the author himself. See appendices Table A.2 (p.118). There is no dose criteria for levels above 5.
The dose level of C is a reference value from the Chernobyl accident.
[http://mext-atm.jst.go.jp/atomica/index.html]

site risk. The Tokaimura criticality accident in Japan was classified as level 4. However, the impression on society-at-large differed considerably. Here, attention is paid to the classification of accidents according to the physical impact on the public. Even if the nuclear event is considered to be an accident in the plant, it is sometimes classified as an extraordinary phenomenon according to this international scale.

1.8 Field Investigations of Nuclear Hazards

One remarkable characteristic of nuclear disaster is the long-term radioactive pollution of the environment due to fission products and plutonium with long half-lives. Nuclear test explosions and accidents that occurred in the last century remain nuclear hazards for local populations even in the present century.

Was the level of radiation exposure and nuclear pollution around nuclear weapon test site acceptable for the local population? Many cases remain unclear even in the 21st century since all the tests conducted were military and secret. Was there no exposure on the population around a plutonium production factory? How do the annual dose and radiological conditions change after the Chernobyl accident?

The author has been investigating dosimetry for the populations at hazard in order to obtain answers to these questions since 1995. A portable laboratory system weighing just 15 kg has been developed for overseas investigations. It contains several small radiation detectors, a GPS navigator, a notebook size

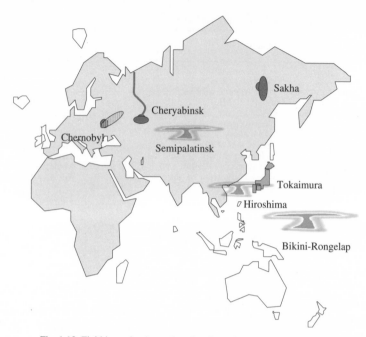

Fig. 1.12 Field investigations of nuclear hazards conducted by the author.

computer and other equipment. This system enables *in-situ* measurements of not only the environment but also of the human body, including whole-body activity measurements. There exists a Russian mobile laboratory in which several radiation detectors are installed in an automobile. The author's system is much smaller. A scientist can bring this portable laboratory anywhere in the world by

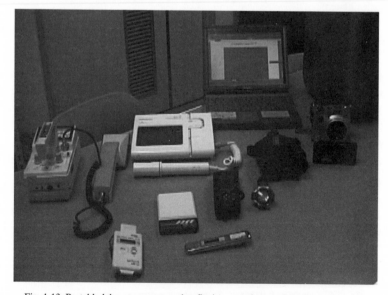

Fig. 1.13 Portable laboratory system that fits in a travel case of airplane cabin size.

boat, plane or car. Residents in nuclear hazard areas often feel fear of radiation exposure. With this system the author can give them the results of measurement immediately.

Hazards investigated in this volume include the Mayak plutonium complex in Russia, the area around the Semipalatinsk nuclear weapons test site in Kazakhstan, Rongelap Atoll effected by USA thermonuclear tests in Bikini, industrial nuclear explosion in Sakha, the control zone after the Chernobyl accident and the residential area around the Tokaimura criticality accident. The first finding in the author's investigation includes several dangerous radiation exposures in the past. The second finding is decrease in radiological pollution and freedom from radiation exposure of populations residing near hazardous areas. This monograph reviews not only recovery from radiation hazards but also the revival of Hiroshima as a society in the final chapter.

Table 1.3 Equipment included in the portable laboratory system

Device	Description or unit of measurement	Model
GPS	Global position	Magellan GPS3000
Distance	Meter	Lytespeed 400
Gamma survey	Micro sievert per hour Sv, Sv/h	Aloka PDR-101 Polomaster PM1209
Gamma dosimeter	Micro sievert	Aloka PDM-101
Alpha and beta counter	Counts per minute	Aloka TCS-352
NaI (Tl) sectrometer	Cs-137 (Bq)	Hamamatsu C-3475
Notebook type computer		Sony PCG-322B

REFERENCES

1. Science Council of Japan, *Investigation Reports of the Atomic Bomb Disaster* (1953) (in Japanese)
2. W. C. Roesch, ed., *US-Japan Joint Reassessment of Atomic Bomb Radiation Dosimetry in Hiroshima and Nagasaki, Final report,* Hiroshima, Radiation Effects Research Foundation Vol. 1 (1987)
3. I. Shigematsu et al., ed. *Effects of A-bomb Radiation on the Human Body*, Harwood Academic Publishers, Bunkodo Co., Ltd., Tokyo (1995)
4. M. L. Gritzner, W. A. Woolson, *US-Japan Joint Reassessment of Atomic Bomb Radiation Dosimetry in Hiroshima and Nagasaki, Final report*, Hiroshima, Radiation Effects Research Foundation, Vol. 2, 342 (1987)
5. N. Kamada et al., *J. Hiroshima Med. Assoc.*, **51**, 355 (1998) (in Japanese)
6. S. Glasstone, P. J. Dolan, *The Effects of Nuclear Weapons*, United States Department of Defense and the Energy Research and Development Administration (1977)
7. SCOPE59, *Nuclear Test Explosions*, John Wiley & Sons, Chichester (2000)
8. United Nations Scientific Committee on the Effects of Atomic Radiation, *Sources and Effects of Ionizing Radiation*, United Nations, New York (1993)

2

Pollution around the Mayak Plutonium Production Complex

Mayak, a production plant producing weapons-grade plutonium in the former USSR, was responsible for nuclear waste pollution severely affecting inhabitants of the surrounding area. The internal exposure of the residents to strontium-90 (Sr-90) by contamination of the Techa River is a disaster unrivaled elsewhere in the world. In this chapter, we report mainly on the local investigations conducted in April and May 2000. The disaster was studied not only by field investigation but also by the Russian Institutes of Radiation Hygiene, Research Institute for Industrial and Marine Medicine and the Urals Research Center for Radiation Medicine.[1,2] Radiological fieldwork was carried out in one settlement along the Techa River and in two other settlements of the Southern Ural Mountains region in collaboration with local scientists, governments and residents.

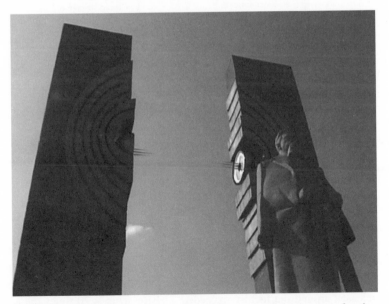

Fig. 2.1 A statue of Igor Kurchatov, the leader of research and development of nuclear weapons in Chelyabinsk City, USSR.

2.1 A Brief History of the Radiological Hazards in the Southern Urals

In 1949, the production of weapons-grade plutonium in the USSR started in the Southern Ural Mountains. This was the first nuclear plant in the USSR. Lavrenti Beria, state minister of domestic affairs, was put in change of construction. The Semipalatinsk nuclear weapons test site is 1400 km east of Mayak, which is located 60 km northwest of Chelyabinsk City.

This facility consisted of three main components, a reactor plant, a radiochemical facility and a waste storage facility (Fig. 2.2).[3] Four radiological disasters originated in Mayak: the discharge of 1.0×10^{17} Bq of liquid waste into the Techa River between 1949 and 1956, an explosion in the storage facility of radioactive wastes at Kyshtym in 1957 (called the Kyshtym accident), which led to the formation of the East Urals Radioactive Trace (EURT) as a result of the dispersion of 7.4×10^{16} Bq into the atmosphere and the resuspension of 2.2×10^{13} Bq with dry silt from the shore of Lake Karachay during a heavy thunderstorm in 1967, and gaseous-aerosol releases of 2.1×10^{16} Bq, mainly during the first decade of operation at Mayak.

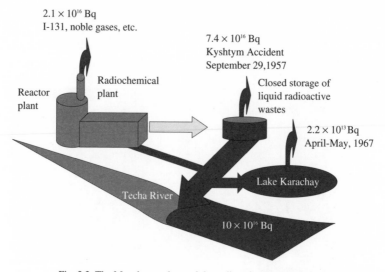

Fig. 2.2 The Mayak complex and the radioactive waste released.

On January 27, 1993, the Russian government released the first official report on the actual state of radioactive pollution in the Urals district. According to the Russian Cabinet Minister Conference Caucus, the total amount of radioactive waste released around the factory exceeded 37 EBq. This is 20 times the amount released in the Chernobyl nuclear accident. Approximately 450,000 individuals were exposed to radiation. Of 50,000 individuals exposed to higher doses 1000 became ill. Radioactivity spread mainly in the three states of Chelyabinsk, Kurgan and Sverdrovsk around the factory. In response, the Russian Cabinet Minister Conference Caucus decided to provide compensation for the victims and to develop a plan to monitor pollution from Mayak.

Inhabitants along the Techa River used the river as a source of drinking water. The long-term investigation of health effects on the residents shows that the risk of death from leukemia and other cancers increased with dose.

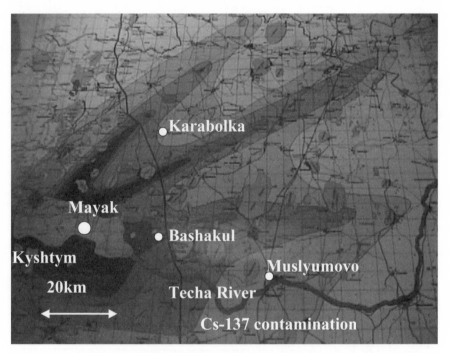

Fig. 2.3 Map of the areas around Mayak.
[From Kunashak Administration, Chelyabinsk Oblast, Russia]

Twenty-five percent of the nuclear fission material which flowed into the Techa River was Sr-90 and cesium-137 (Cs-137), both with a long half-life. Over 95 percent of radioactive waste was disposed of between 1950 and 1951. Radioactivity in water decreases as it flows away from the source. The intake of radioactive material among the people living upstream and midstream of the river was higher than among those living downstream. The polluted river became a source of secondary pollution in cows, milk and agricultural products.

About 7,500 inhabitants who lived upstream and midstream of the Techa River were evacuated between 1956 and 1960. In the meantime, about 2,000 inhabitants were exposed to radiation together with fallout from the Kyshtym accident, which occurred in 1957. Moreover, inhabitants living within 60 km of Mayak were also affected by the gaseous radioactivity that leaked regularly from the facility.

Wide-area monitoring of the residents along the Techa River began in 1951. In these investigations, the long-term effects on the human body due to pollution by radioactive materials with a long half-life were examined. A special data base for the protection of residents from radiation has been created by the Urals Research Center for Radiation Medicine. The main characteristic was internal exposure to Sr-90. Because calcium and strontium are in the same chemical family, strontium accumulates in bone and teeth. The β-rays from this Sr-90 irradiated bone marrow for a long period of time.

2.2 Radiological Investigations in Various Settlements

2.2.1   Muslyumovo (Techa River 1949-1956)

The Techa River, which is located upstream of the Ob' River, flows into the Kara Sea in the north after changing names several times (Iset, Tobol and Irtysh). Therefore, nuclear waste matter was carried from the Urals into the sea in the north. Muslyumovo is the only village that remained after the other villages were evacuated due to pollution of the river.

Radiation measurements were conducted in the floodplain 180 m from the iron railroad bridge that passes the village. The radiological contamination was localized in the Techa River. The radiation level (Cs-137 of 0.6 MBq/m² and dose rate of 1 μSv/h) on the floodplain was the same as that in the strict control zone of the Chernobyl accident. It was ten times higher than that in a grass field far from the river's edge.

Beta counts of grass samples from the floodplain indicated 3.1 cpm/g. Cows ate grass on the floodplain and drank water at the river. However, no clear beta count was detected in their milk.

The radiation was 24 kBq/m² and 0.05 μSv/h in a forest of white birch behind a hospital. This is not a level of concern.

The average dose rate during a seven-hour stay in this village in 2000 was 0.07 μSv/h, which was within the normal range.

Radioactivity in carp was measured at the request of fishermen. The whole-body burdens were Cs-137 of 11 kBq/kg and β counts of 359 cpm (75 cpm/g for scales, 11 cpm/g for backbone, not detectable for other organs). Fish was a major source of food for the village.

Beta counts on teeth and forehead was carried out on nine villagers who volunteered or requested it. Remarkable counts of 733 and 467 cpm on teeth were observed for two villagers born in 1946 and 1950, respectively. Low counts were detected in other parts of the body. Strontium accumulated in bone or tooth and continued to radiate β-rays long term. Because this radiation cannot penetrate a sheet of thin metal, it is difficult to measure β-rays from Sr-90 in backbone. Since teeth are exposed and therefore more accessible, they were easier to measure.

Others who were not born near the period of massive release did not show remarkable β counts. The villagers now drink well water. A fence was constructed on the riverside, but the grazing cows drank water at the river and ingested grass on the banks. Milk in the village did not show remarkable β counts. However, the

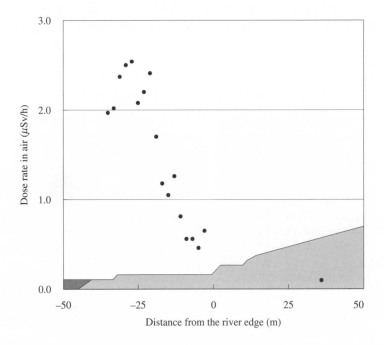

Fig. 2.4 Gamma dose rate on the floodplain of the Techa River in Muslyumovo village in 2000.

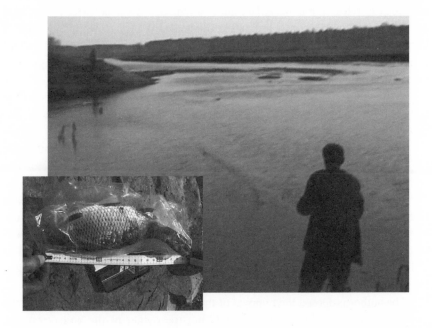

Fig. 2.5 A fisherman and carp in the Techa River.

villager probably drank polluted milk in 1950-1951 without realizing it.

The present β observation was consistent with Sr-90 in the data base of URCRM. Body burden of Cs-137 for three residents was less than the detectable limit (20 Bq/kg).

Measurement of a large horn of an elk which was hunted in Muslyumovo showed a β count of 98 cpm. It probably drank water from the Techa River.

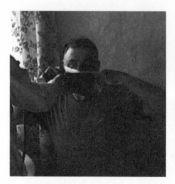 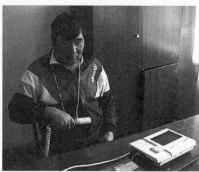

Fig. 2.6. Beta counting on front teeth (left) and whole-body counting of Cs-137.

2.2.2   Bashakul (Lake Karachay Trace 1967)

The village of Bashakul was polluted by fallout due to the large amount of radioactivity released into the environment when Lake Karachay dried up in 1967.

The radiation in a forest in Bashakul indicated 0.1 μSv/h with Cs-137 of 75 kBq/m². The yard of a kindergarten showed a nearly normal level of 0.05 μSv/h with Cs-137 of 16 kBq/m². The average dose rate during a seven-hour stay in this village was 0.07 μSv/h.

WBC of Cs-137 and β count on teeth were carried out on seven residents. The body burden of radio cesium was less than the detectable limit for all of them. The maximum β count was 53 cpm.

For some reason, soil on the ceilings of houses was contaminated, indicating Cs-137 of 1.6 MBq/m² and a β count of 2.6 kcpm in one house (No. 19). The highest dose rate was 1.7 μSv/h in the room.

The 51-year-old owner of the house had been evacuated from the Techa riverside to this village with his parents in 1956. The government built this house for them. He explained that soil on the ceiling had been laid in 1956. This was before the Karachay disaster and the Kyshtym accident. Where did this radioactive soil come from? We can not imagine such contaminated soil from the Techa. Other homes in the area also demonstrated radioactivity.

The author proposed the removal of the contaminated soil from ceiling to the local government, which agreed to try, but the owner of the house refused. Scientific proposals do not always work in society.

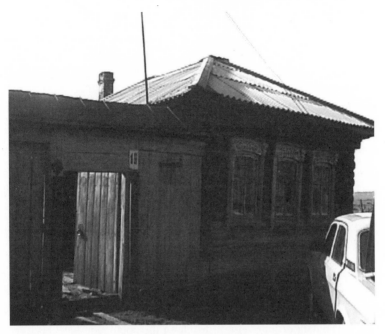

Fig. 2.7 A radiologically contaminated house in Bashakul.

2.2.3   Karabolka (EURT 1957)

Tatarskaya (T) Karabolka was located in an area suffering from radioactive fallout from the Kyshtym Accident in 1957. The neighboring village of Maraya (M) Karabolka was evacuated just after the accident. However, no such intervention was made for T-Karabolka. Under these circumstances, a field investigation was requested by an individual whose home village was T-Karabolka.

The radiation in a forest near T-Karabolka was 0.06–0.07 μSv/h with Cs-137 of 22 kBq/m². The author conducted measurements on the floodplain of a small river in the village at the request of a woman who feared radioactive contamination. The dose rate was found to be quite normal at 0.05 μSv/h with Cs-137 of 4.2 kBq/m².

Bata count measurement on teeth, forehead and the back of hand was carried out on six residents of T-Karabolka. The maximum values were 19, 46 and 32 cpm respectively.

The radiation in a forest near M-Karabolka was 0.05 μSv/h with Cs-137 of 31 kBq/m². The radiation was almost the same level as that for the forest near T-Karabolka.

Table 2.1 Summary of radiological conditions in the Chelyabinsk region in 2000.

Site	Classification	Specification	Cs-137 (kBq/m^2)	γ dose rate (μSv/h)	net β count rate (cpm)
BK01	Forest	East	73	0.097	53
BK02	Roof	House 19	1630	nm*	2580
BK03	Yard	Kindergarten	15.6	0.050	41
BK04	Forest	West	76.1	0.096	62
ML01	Bank	Waterworks	116	0.118	164
ML02	Forest	Hospital	24.4	0.047	29
ML03	Floodplain	180m Bridge	563	1.040	314
ML04	Grass Field	180m Bridge	52	0.097	14
ML05	Grass Field	Administration	8.8	0.032	31
ML06	Floodplain	Mill	445	0.550	294
TK01	Forest	West	21.5	0.062	42
TK02	Floodplain	Bridge	4.2	0.050	50
TK03	Forest	East	21.5	0.071	44
MK04	Forest	North	31.1	0.045	21

BK: Bashakul, ML: Muslyumovo, TK: Tatarskaya Karabolka
*nm: not measured

2.3 Urals Research Center for Radiation Medicine

Nuclear accidents have resulted in hazardous radioactive exposure of the general population. The data of long-term research on the population have been recorded at the Urals Research Center for Radiation Medicine (URCRM) in Chelyabinsk.[4] The research results have been summarized in a data base.

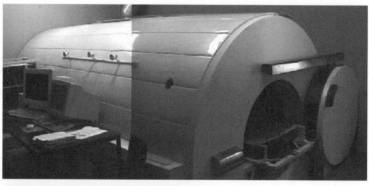

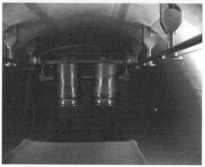

Fig. 2.8 Whole-body counter of Sr-90 in URCRM.

An autopsy program of strontium 90 radioactivity analysis in human bone samples was continued until 1993. More than 7,500 analyses of samples obtained from 5400 autopsies of Urals residents were conducted.

In earlier investigations, those who were exposed to radiation could not be effectively examined. However, since 1959, β-ray counting on the front teeth made it possible to investigate radiation exposure on the living. Since 1974, the residents of the Techa riverside have been measured for body burden of Sr-90 and Cs-137 using the whole-body counter.

The data base MAIN contains individual data on 90,000 individuals exposed to radiation on the banks of the Techa River and/or in the territories covered by the EURT. A remarkable observation was the internal exposure to Sr-90 for the residents living along the Techa River.[4,5] The maximum values of Sr-90 body burden were reported to be 80–4 kBq for adult residents of the upper and mid-Techa region between 1952 and 1990. More than half showed red bone marrow (RBW) dose between 0.1 and 0.5 Gy due to Sr-89, -90 and Cs-137. Doses due to Pu-239, -240 were provisionally estimated to be 1.5–2.5 mSv for RBW and 10–15 mSv for bone surface.

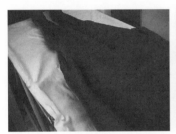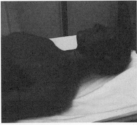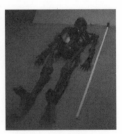

Fig. 2.9 Sr-90 whole-body phantom developed by the Research and Technical Center in St. Petersburg.

2.3.1 Strontium-90 in the Body

Figure 2.10 shows the annual change in Sr-90 body burden of residents of the Techa region. The average level decreased to single-digit values over a period of 40 years. The level of the Techa residents is remarkably high by more than two orders of magnitude compared with residents in other global fallout areas.

The Sr-90 body burdens decrease with distance from the source of radioactivity leakage. The maximum body burden in each village was proportional to the Sr-90 concentration in river water. This was evidence that the residents ingested Sr-90 from water in the river. In 1951 it was prohibited to obtain water supply from the river and inhabitants upstream were relocated. Those living in the lower part of the river were relocated after 1956.

The levels of Sr-90 in tooth and bone differ by age. Teeth start growing in infancy. As for the growth rate of the bone, it is greatest in 15-year-old boys. Fig. 2.11 shows a large difference between these two organs. The enamel of the front

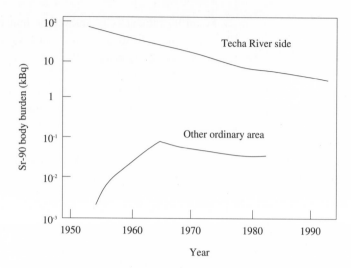

Fig. 2.10 Sr-90 body burdens for adult residents of the upper and mid-Techa regions.
[Reproduced with permission from M.O. Degteva, V.P. Kozheurov, E.I. Tolstykh, *Radiation Protection Dosimetry*, **79**, 155 (1998) ©Oxford University Press]

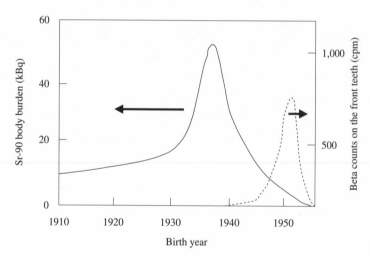

Fig. 2.11 Average values of Sr-90 body burden (solid line) and tooth b count rate (dashed line) among Muslyumovo residents in 1976.
[Reproduced with permission from M.O. Degteva, V.P. Kozheurov, E.I. Tolstykh, *Radiation Protection Dosimetry*, **79**, 155 (1998) ©Oxford University Press]

teeth is formed in a very short period of time while the metabolism of the enamel is slow. This results in a remarkable peak of Sr-90 intake in infancy.

2.3.2   Cesium and Plutonium

The body burden of Cs-137 for Techa residents in the period 1974-1985 was about twice the global level. However, as a result of fallout from the Chernobyl accident in 1986, the body burden of the residents reached a peak in 1987. Since the biological half-life of Cs-137 is 100 days, dose reconstruction for this nuclide is difficult.

There was no special program for measuring plutonium-239, -240 (Pu-239, -240) for the Techa River cohort. However, an investigation of approximately 7,000 samples from 680 autopsies of the residents in the Chelyabinsk region was implemented by the First Branch of the Institute of Biophysics in Moscow. The body burden of the plutonium decreased rapidly with distance from Mayak, indicating that plutonium intake was the result of gaseous aerosol releases.

2.4 Summary

Enormous environmental pollution was caused by nuclear waste around plutonium production facilities for the development of nuclear weapons in the former USSR. The Ministry of Emergency Situations of the Russian Federation has conducted administrative work investigating and seeking countermeasures.[6,7]

A remarkable nuclear disaster in the Southern Ural Mountains was caused by discharges of 1.0×10^{17} Bq of liquid wastes into the Techa River between 1949 and 1956. Radioactive strontium accumulated in the bone of residents. More than half the inhabitants suffered doses of between 0.1 and 0.5 Gy in red bone marrow due to Sr-89, -90 and Cs-137. β-Rays were also detected on the front teeth of some residents who born around 1950 due to the long biological half-life of Sr-90. The residual radioactivity was localized in the floodplain of the Techa River where the level of radiation was of the same order as that found in the zone of strict control after the Chernobyl nuclear accident.

Radioactive pollution occurred due to an explosion in a radioactive waste storage facility at Kyshtym in 1957 and the resuspension of nuclear waste from the shore of Lake Karachay in 1967. The village of Bashakul, which had been polluted by fallout from Lake Karachay, showed low risk γ-dose rate of 0.1 μSv/h or less, with Cs-137 of 75 kBq/m^2 in 2000.

The Russian Federation has accumulated much information from many experiences and data on radiation protection and hygiene for the public from the nuclear accidents and disasters that occurred during the period of the former Soviet Union. Several institutes, including the Institute of Radiation Hygiene, the Urals Research Center for Radiation Medicine and the Institute of Biophysics have been taking charge of scientific investigations into these nuclear hazards.

Data from long-term research on the population around the Mayak plutonium production facility have been recorded at the URCRM in Chelyabinsk. Data bases have been created for dose reconstruction and risk assessment.

Three settlements were investigated using a portable laboratory system developed by the author in 2000. Remarkable β-ray counts were observed in the teeth of residents born in Muslyumovo between 1946 and 1950, consistent with the information in the β base of URCRM. Radiological conditions except those for the region of the Techa River were acceptable from the viewpoint of radiation hygiene in this limited investigation.

REFERENCES

1. J. Takada, *Radiation Science*, **43**, 34 (2000) (in Japanese)
2. J. Takada, V. Sharov, Yu. O. Konstantinov, P.V. Ramzaev, G. Moroz, A. Kovtum, M. Hoshi, N.G. Bougrov, H.A. Shishkina, L. Premyslova, N. Shagina, M.O. Degteva, *Proceedings Mission for the Study of Radiation Protection and Hygiene for Residents Around the Mayak Plutonium Production Facilities in Russia 2000.* International Workshop on Distribution and Speciation of Radionuclides in the Environment, Rokkasho-mura, Japan, October 11-13, 2000
3. M.O. Degteva, *Environmental Dose Reconstruction for the Urals Population* (Private communication) (2000)
4. A.V. Akleyev, M.F. Kisselyov, ed., *Medical-biological and Ecological Impacts of Radioactive Contamination of the Techa River*, Russian Federation Health Ministry, Federal Office of Medical-Biological Issues and Emergencies, Urals Research Center for Radiation Medicine, Moscow (2000)
5. M.O. Degteva, V.P. Kozheurov, E.I. Tolstykh, *Radiation Protection Dosimetry*, **79**, 155 (1998)
6. Technical Disaster Center, *Administration of the Chelyabinsk Region, Radiation Monitoring Zone Affected by Mayak* (1996) (in Russian)
7. V.Ya. Voznyak, V.V. Panteleyev, *Basic Principles of Federal Policy for Rehabilitation of Territories and Residents Exposed to Radiation*, International Congress on Radiation Protection (IRPA 9) in Vienna, Austria, April 14-19 (1996)

3

Semipalatinsk Nuclear Tests

The main nuclear weapon test sites of the former Soviet Union were located in Semipalatinsk and Novaya Zemlya. The total numbers of test and output were 969 and 285 megatons. The Semipalatinsk nuclear test site in Kazakhstan has been opened to foreign scientists to investigate the radiation hazard since 1991, after the fall of the Soviet Union. The author's team has been studying radiation effects, mainly dosimetry, for the population around the test site in Semipalatinsk since 1995. In this chapter, we report mainly data on retrospective dose and present environmental radiological levels.[1,2]

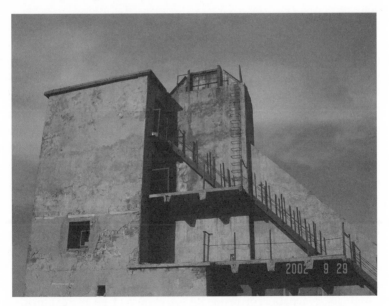

Fig. 3.1 Tower used for measurements of nuclear weapon effects near ground zero.

3.1 A Brief History of the Semipalatinsk Nuclear Test Site

A total of 459 nuclear tests were conducted by the former USSR between 1949 and 1989 at the Semipalatinsk Nuclear Test Site (SNTS) in Kazakhstan, including 87 atmospheric, 26 ground and 346 underground explosions.[3] The total release of the energy equivalent of trinitrotoluene (TNT) of about 18 Mt was 1100 times that of the Hiroshima atomic bomb. This output is 6% of all the nuclear explosions in the USSR. A village and a city are located close to the test site, and the inhabitants of the area suffered serious health effects.

The first nuclear weapon test in the USSR was conducted at the SNTS on August 29, 1949. It is said to that this first nuclear bomb was a copy of the Nagasaki bomb made according to plans stolen from the U.S. by a spy. The explosion occurred 38 m above the ground, and the energy output was equivalent to 22 kilotons of TNT. An explosion which covers the surface of the earth is classified as a surface explosion. For area residents, this type of nuclear explosion is the most dangerous in terms of radiation exposure. Two hours after this nuclear test, a huge radioactive cloud formed over Dolon and other villages more than 70 km from the epicenter.[1]

This first explosion is considered to be the most dangerous nuclear bomb for the population near the nuclear test site for the following reasons.[4] The explosion was detonated on the ground under rain and strong wind conditions of up to 75 m/s. Moreover, villages downwind were not evacuated. Under these conditions, very high radioactive contamination occurred and inhabitants were exposed to the radiation.

On August 12, 1953, the first thermonuclear weapon was exploded in the same place as the first nuclear explosion of 1949. This occurred at 50 m above ground and the energy output was equivalent to 400 kt of TNT. The residents in the direction of Karaul village were evacuated for three days after this explosion.[5] The radioactive cloud passed through Karaul in three hours due to a wind speed of 40–45 km/m^2, which was higher than expected. It was said that 191 villagers who did not evacuate in time were exposed to radiation.

On January 15, 1965, a thermonuclear bomb equivalent to 140 kilotons of TNT was exploded 200 m underground in the eastern part of the test site. The official reason given for this explosion was the construction of a dam for peaceful use. As a result of this experiment, there now exists a lake, which is known by the inhabitants of the area as "Atomic Lake."

Nuclear weapon explosions were carried out at the Semipalatinsk test site until 1989 without any formal information provided for the population. The test site, called the Polygon, was located on the western side of Semipalatinsk State. The population of the state was 410,000 in 1949 and 750,000 in 1962. There was no preliminary evacuation of residents for almost of all the explosion tests. Therefore, the residents downwind were exposed to radiation by fallout. As far as is known, evacuation was conducted only for the first thermonuclear test. The history of nuclear disasters in Kazakhstan started due to the nuclear weapon development by the former USSR in this way.

Various measurements were conducted by the military during the tests both within and outside the test site. They secretly investigated dosimetry and health

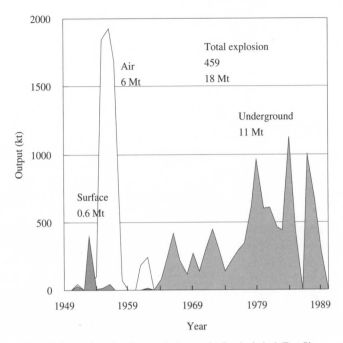

Fig. 3.2 Dynamics of nuclear explosions at the Semipalatinsk Test Site.
[From Russian Federal Nuclear Center- VNIIEF, 1996]

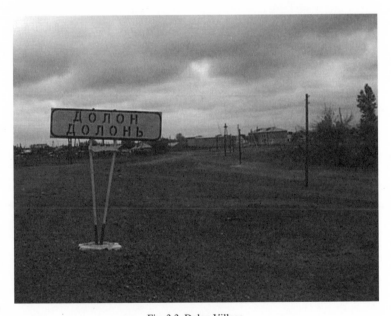

Fig. 3.3 Dolon Village.

effects on the population. After Kazakhstan gained independence in 1991, these data were opened to the public. There are some residential areas where the dose reaches several sieverts.

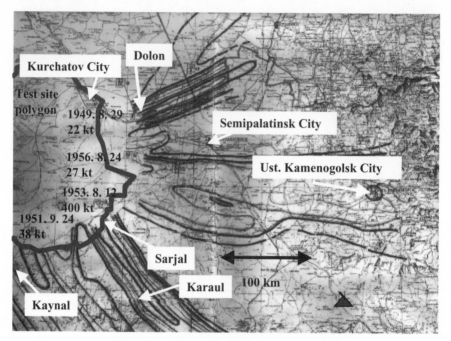

Fig. 3.4 Dose map for some nuclear explosions around SNTS.
[From *Kazakhstan Republic Iso-dose Map* (1964)]

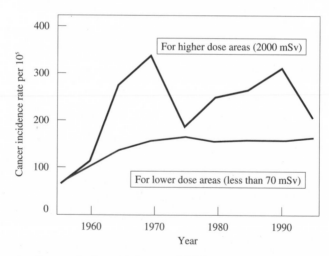

Fig. 3.5 Dynamics of cancers for the population around SNTS.
[Reproduced with permission from B.I. Gusev, *Tumor Incidence Among Inhabitants of Some Districts in the Semipalatinsk Region Exposed after Nuclear Testing at the Test Ground, Proc. of the 2nd Hiroshima International Symposium, Hiroshima*, 153-194 (1996)]

Dr. B.I. Gusev of the Kazakh Scientific Research Institute of Radiation and Ecology and Dr. V.F. Stepanenko of the Russian Academy of Medical Science each reported the doses of the area residents. The value obtained by the former is higher than that obtained by the latter. As for the dose in Dolon, even the official

Russian report was 1.6 Gy.[5,6]

An oncological study of the population in the Semipalatinsk region has been carried out since 1956. The cancer incidence rate increased rapidly after 1960 and reached the maximum value of 400 per 100,000 in 1970.[7]

Up to 1995, none of the reports concerning the effects of radiation on residents near the SNTS based on data provided by the Defense Department of the former USSR[5,6] used direct experimental data concerning the effective equivalent dose. They just measured some doses in particular settlements after some nuclear explosions. Therefore the value does not indicate the accumulation of dose from all explosions between 1949 and 1989. High dose values have been reported for some settlements, as shown in Table 3.1. However, there are large discrepancies in the values reported before and after the independence of the Republic of Kazakhstan.

Table. 3.1 Reported values of total dose for populations from Russia and Kazakhstan

Area	R/S	External plus internal dose (Sv)	
		Russia	Kazakhstan
Abaisky	R	0.10	0.11
Beskaragaisky	R	0.05	1.95
Jana-Seminsky	R	0.00	0.21
Dolon	S	1.60	4.47
Karaul	S	0.37	0.88
Kainar	S	0.24	0.68
Sarjal	S	0.20	2.46
Semipalatinsk	S	0.01	—

Russia: A.H. Tsyb, V.F. Stepanenko 1989[6]
Kazakhstan: B.I. Gusev 1993[5]
R: Region S: Settlement

3.2 Thermoluminescence Dosimetry for Exposed Bricks

The technique of thermoluminescence dosimetry (TLD), which were successfully applied in the dosimetry for the Hiroshima and Nagasaki nuclear bombs,[8,9] enabled us to evaluate the accumulated external γ-ray doses of all the nuclear explosions at specific places around the SNTS. The TLD technique is well established not only for instantaneous exposure to the nuclear bombs dropped on Hiroshima and Nagasaki[10] but also for prolonged exposure to natural radiation, which is used in dating.[11] Moreover, this technique was applicable for dosimetry studies of radioactive fallout as shown in studies of the Chernobyl Accident.[12,13] The author and his team applied TLD to a dosimetry study of the local population in the Semipalatinsk nuclear test area.

We attempted dose reconstruction for the local populations based on the results of a study using the thermoluminescence technique on brick samples from several settlements in 1995, 1996 and 1997. The areas investigated include Dolon and other villages, Semipalatinsk City and Ust-Kamenogorsk City.

We sampled bricks from the surface of the outer walls of buildings mainly in

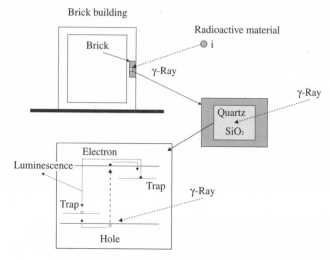

Fig. 3.6 Principle of TLD.

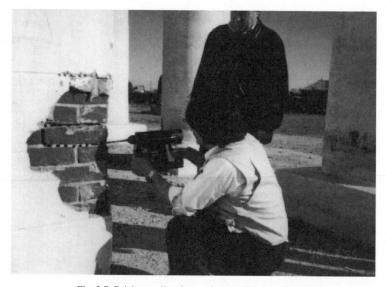

Fig. 3.7 Brick sampling from a former church at Dolon.

three settlements around the SNTS. Two of them were Semipalatinsk City and Ust-Kamenogorsk City. They were located 100 km and 270 km from the boundary of the SNTS. The previously reported doses for these areas were not so clear compared with those for other small settlements.

The third area examined was the village of Dolon and other small settlements. Dolon, which is located 55 km from the boundary of the SNTS, was one of the settlements indicating the highest dose in a former report.[5] Each coordinate of the sampling sites was measured by GPS Navigator.

The experimental procedure for the estimation of external γ-ray dose by TLD has been described previously.[8,14] The quartz inclusion method was applied to sample preparations.[14] The surface of brick samples was removed in thicknesses ranging from 5 to 10 mm. The next 20 mm of the brick was used for sample preparation. High temperature analysis of thermoluminescence was applied using the TLD device with a single photon counting system (Daybreak Nuclear and Medical Systems, Inc., 1100 TL system).

We measured the *in-situ* γ-ray dose rate at the surface of the sampling point using a pocket survey meter (Aloka PDR-101), in which a CsI (Tl) ($20 \times 25 \times 15$ mm) detector was installed. We used these data for the estimation of natural γ-ray exposure for bricks in TLD analysis. The β-ray internal dose rate for quartz grain was measured for each brick sample in the laboratory. Measurement was conducted by sandwiching CaSO4:Dy TL powder between two disks of brick samples, which were stored in a 10 cm-thick Pb shielding box with N_2 gas,[8] and β counting on the surface of a brick sample (ZnS(Ag) plastic scintillator (Aloka TCS-35, active area, 72 cm²) was performed. The former was done to obtain the absolute value and the latter to obtain the relative value. A clean surface was prepared by cutting each brick sample for β measurements.

The dose component due to α particles originating within the clay matrix was rendered negligible by etching the surface of the quartz. The age of the brick was assumed to be the same as the age of the building.

3.3 External Dose Reconstruction

The number of samples obtained from a building at each location was usually one in the present report. The bricks were obtained from the outer surface of the buildings. The number of brick buildings was very limited, especially in the villages (usually one).

The method of external dose estimation by TLD for brick is summarized in Fig. 3.8. The external dose of free space in air (D_{AirF}) 1 m above the ground surface is assumed to be approximately twice the surface dose (D_{SF}) of a brick-building wall since there is no radioactivity due to the radioactive fallout and cloud contained inside building.

The D_{SF} is estimated using the dose (D_F^*) in the brick due to the radioactive cloud and fallout employing the transmission coefficient (T_{av}) of the brick for γ-rays from fission products, as expressed by eq. (3.1).

$$D_{SF} = D_F^* / T_{av} \tag{3.1}$$

In our study, we applied the transmission coefficient (T_{av} : 0.8–0.7) of bricks for γ-rays of cesium-137 (Cs-137) to the estimate obtained for each sample.

Fission products of Sr (strontium) -91, Sr-92, Zr (zirconium) -97, Ru (ruthenium) -105, I (iodine) -132, I-133, I-134, I-135, La (lanthanum) -140 and La-142 as γ emitters are the main sources of the radioactivity of the external dose on residents living more than several tens of kilometers from the test site, from the

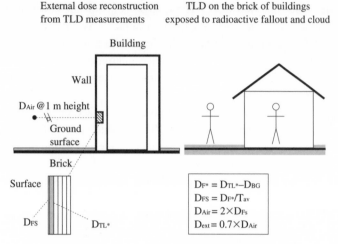

Fig. 3.8 Schematic illustration of dose reconstruction for residents obtained by TLD measurements in brick.

half-life point of view.[16,17] Weighted mean values of γ energy for each nuclide were calculated for γ-rays with intensity per decay of more than 10%. The effective energy of γ-rays from these fallout activities is estimated to be 855 keV as the weighted average of effective γ-ray energy for each nuclide by its dose contribution (3h–7d). The difference in transmission coefficient between the 855 keV γ-ray and 662 keV Cs-137 γ-ray, which is estimated to be about 10%, is acceptable in the present dosimetry study.

This is supported by TLD studies of fallout from atomic power plant accidents. The Monte Carlo calculation for isotropic irradiation from a homogenous source distributed on the ground surface with Cs-137 is consistent with TLD depth profiles for bricks exposed to Chernobyl fallout.[14] Thus, D_F^* can be expressed by the following equation:

$$D_F^* = D_{TL}^* - D_{BG} \tag{3.2}$$

where D_{TL}^* and D_{BG} are the raw values of dose in the brick and natural background dose, respectively. Correction of the measured D_{TL}^* values for supralinearity was less than 10 %.

The external dose (D_{Ext}) for humans is somewhat less than D_{AirF} since they have body shielding and are not always outside. The radiation level indoors is less than that outdoors. The ratio (D_{Ext} /D_{AirF}), which depends on the structure of the building and the inhabitant's lifestyle, is reported to be 0.73[18] or 0.65[19] for nuclear weapon explosions and the Chernobyl accident. We note that no special measures were taken for radiation protection of residents for most of the explosions. Therefore, D_{Ext} /D_{AirF} is likely to be about 0.7, and we estimated D_{Ext} by

$$D_{Ext} = 0.7 \, D_{Air} \tag{3.3}$$

3.4 External Dose to Populations

The external doses are summarized in Table 3.2. The present results of external doses in small settlements such as Dolon and Chagan are consistent with previously reported values. We confirmed the external dose of residents in Dolon due to the radioactive cloud and fallout from the SNT to be at a level of 1 Gy.

Table 3.2 Dose in settlements around the Semipalatinsk Nuclear Test Site

Settlement	Number of site (s)	Dose		
		Dfs (Gy)	Dair (Gy)	Dext (Gy)
Dolon	1	0.71	1.42	0.99
Izvyestka	1	0.30	0.60	0.42
Chagan	1	0.25	0.50	0.35
Semipalatinsk City				
Center of city	3	0.44 ± 0.07	0.89 ± 0.14	0.62 ± 0.10
Other sites	3	BG	BG	BG

BG: Background level
[From J. Takada et al., *J. Radiat. Res.*, **40**, 337 (1999)]

The external doses at a total of six sites of Semipalatinsk City were as high as 0.69 Gy. Three sites in the center of the city exhibited 0.62 ± 0.10 Gy. This is remarkably high compared with the previously reported value, which was 0.004 Sv. Doses at the other three sites were background level.

Such a large discrepancy indicates the need for further investigation. The total number of reported doses after each nuclear explosion was very small compared with the total number of nuclear explosions (459). For example, there were only 21 explosions during the period 1949 to 1965 in an iso-dose line map, as reported by Logachev.[20] Moreover, no information on doses in and around Semipalatinsk City is shown on the map.

Some underground explosions near the ground surface were equal to a surface explosion from the viewpoint of the radioactivity released to the environment. In Sakha, where twelve underground nuclear explosions were conducted between 1974 and 1987, two were actually accidental surface explosions.[21] In the SNTS, a thermonuclear explosion on January 15, 1965, was classified as being underground in the Russian report,[3] even though the explosion, which had an output of 140 kt at a depth of 200 m, produced a crater on the ground surface. Such a nuclear explosion should be classified as a surface explosion.[22] Moreover, the huge amount of radioactive rare gas rising from the surface after underground explosions seems to be the source of radiation exposure.

Additionally, the amount of military data on Semipalatinsk City that were available for dose reconstruction was extremely limited in the calculation for Stepanenko.[6] Therefore, there is much uncertainty in the previously calculated doses. The most important work will be the dose reconstruction based on data of direct measurement of accumulated dose, which does not require any information on radioactive sources.

The external doses at three sites in the center of the city were larger than those in other parts of the city. We also noted a similar dose distribution around Dolon. The distance between Dolon and Chagan is less than 15 km. This similarity may be due to a difference in the local weather conditions or the narrow trajectory of radioactive clouds. Detailed studies of dose distribution in Semipalatinsk City may require more measuring points in the future.

The external doses at seven sites in Ust-Kamenogorsk City were as high as 0.51 Gy. The average value was 0.29 ± 0.17 Gy. The M43 isodose map[18] shows a dose outdoors higher than 0.15 Gy as dose in air for Ust-Kamenogorsk City due to the August 1956 explosion (26 kt at $h = 100$ m).[18]

On the other hand, Loborev reported values between 0.02 and 0.06 Sv as effective dose in the city due to four explosions between 1956 and 1962.[23] This evaluation is inconsistent with the present work and the M43 map.

An individual's dose depends on life-style concerning the time spent outdoors, the structure of the house and so on. In a simple model, the individual stays outdoors with external exposure to radiation in open air, and stays indoors with certain γ-ray dose transmission factors.

$$D_{ext} = a \cdot D_o + b \cdot D_i, \ a + b = 1 \tag{3.4}$$

Here, D_o and D_i are dose outdoors and dose indoors, respectively. The ratio D_i/D_o indicates the γ-ray dose transmission factors. A Russian wooden house indicates about 0.3 for this factor. Coefficients a and b indicate the ratio of time spent outdoors and indoors, respectively.

In Table 3.3, calculation results for settlements around SNTS are summarized for various a values in the case of a wooden house with transmission factor of 0.3. The individual dose should be dose with b values of between 1 and 0.

Table 3.3 External doses with varying a values in the case of a wooden house

| Settlement | External dose (mGy) | | | | |
| | Percentage of time spent outdoors (%) | | | | |
	In air	100	0	33	50
Dolon	1420	1164	349	618	757
Chagan	500	410	123	218	267
Isvyostka	600	492	148	261	320
Semipalatinsk City	0-980	0-804	0-244	0-432	0-529
	Av. 445	365	109	194	237
Ust-Kamenogorsk City	47-679	39-557	12-167	20-296	25-362
	Av. 376	308	92	164	200

Wooden house with 30 % transmittance for γ-rays.
Self body shielding of 0.82

People living in rural areas spend longer time outdoors than those living in the city. Much agricultural work is done in Kazakhstan. Multistory buildings in the city have a lower value of γ-ray dose transmission factor than the 0.3 for wooden houses. This may be equal to or less than 0.1.

3.5 Present Status of Radiation in and around Test Sites

Remarkable environmental radiation has been observed only in the test site called the Polygon in our field investigation since 1995. The Polygon was not our main object since no one lived there during the testing period. Therefore there was little data in our work on the test site till 2000. However, since September 11, 2001, terrorism using portable nuclear weapons has become a realistic risk in the city.

Environmental radiation monitoring outside Polygon is very important for radiation hygiene for the Kazakhstan population. Therefore, we did radiation measurements over a wide area. Fortunately, we have not detected any remarkably high radiation due to residual radioactivity from nuclear explosion tests. All the data outside the test site showed a dose rate equal to or less than 0.1 μSv/h.

The radiation level around Atomic Lake, which was created by a crater explosion of 140 kt on January 15, 1965, was still high in 1995. The place is in the zone-II neighborhood of the east boundary of the SNTS. An iron fence was set up around Polygon, and entrance was limited to several places. The diameter and depth of the crater were 400 m and 100 m respectively. The maximum γ dose rate was 21 μSv/h at the edge of the lake in 1995. The α particle counting survey around the crater showed very low counts of several cpm even though there was remarkably high plutonium contamination. We found 159 cpm at only one site in 1999. Counting of α particles is difficult due to very low transmission.

The author and his team visited ground zero (N 50, 26', 16", E 77, 48, 46) in 2001 and 2002. This was marked with a metal flag with the word for epicenter in Russian. Three nuclear explosions, the first plutonium bomb (22 kt, $h = 30$ m, August 29, 1949), the second bomb (38 kt, $h = 30$ m, September 24, 1951) and the first thermonuclear weapon (400 kt, $h = 50$ m, August 12, 1953), were conducted within the area of the polygon by the former USSR. Since the fireball radius can be estimated to be 190–600 m for the three explosions, these were classified as surface nuclear explosions. We found many melted stones and stones with air bubbles in a wide area around ground zero (Fig. 3.9).

Gamma radiation still showed a high level of 10–50 μSv/h at ground zero even in 2002. This is quite different from Hiroshima and Nagasaki where the nuclear explosion (15–20 kt) occurred in the air. The hypocenters in Japan showed radiation of 0.1 μSv/h at the end of the 20th century. The reason for this difference resides in the origin of the residual radioactivity at ground zero. In a surface explosion, the main component is fission products and trans uranium while an explosion in air involves neutron-induced radio nuclides. The latter decay much faster than the former. Therefore, explosions of portable nuclear weapons in a city will show prolonged radiation at ground zero.

The radiation distribution around the epicenter was anisotropic, related to the wind directions at the time of explosion. Residual radiation was observed along

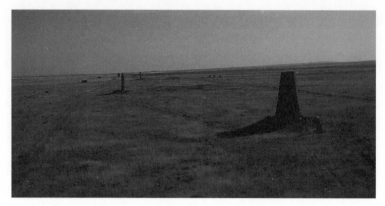

Fig. 3.9 Near ground zero of the first nuclear weapon test. Several concrete towers for measurements of weapon effects remained in 2002. Sampling there was not permitted probably in order to preserve the historic spot.
[Photo courtesy of Mr. N. Fujiyasu]

the trajectory of the fallout.

In 2002 the author and his team investigated another ground zero site in zone I with a guide of the National Nuclear Center (NNC). There were four craters with diameters between 30 and 60 m (Fig. 3.10). This zone was quite different from the other nuclear hazard sites in the author's experience. The α components of radiations were remarkably high.

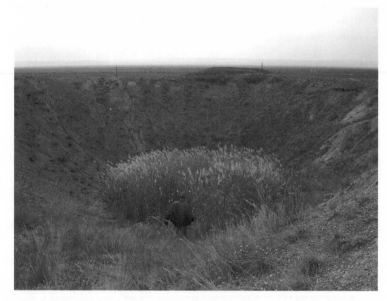

Fig. 3.10 A mysterious small-scale nuclear explosion crater with a diameter of 30 m.

We investigated one of them (N: 50 22' 26", E 77 48' 49"). The area within a radius of 200 m exhibited α count rates of more than 10 cpm with a maximum of

1800 cpm. On the other hand, the γ dose rate was 1.5–3.0 μSv/h, where Cs-137 was on the order of 1 MBq/m^2 maximum.

A crater with a diameter of 30 m and depth of 10 m suggests an explosion with a yield of less than 1 kt. This is less than 1/100 of the yield of the explosion of Atomic Lake. However, there was a much greater level of α emitters in this smaller explosion, suggesting high plutonium contamination. There were three other craters with diameters of 40–60 m in the vicinity. Therefore, this was not a failed test but may have involved a special weapon (Figs. 3.11 and 3.12).

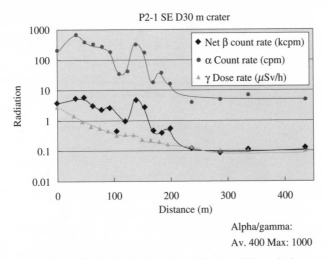

Alpha/gamma:
Av. 400 Max: 1000

Fig. 3.11 Radiation distribution in the southeast direction of the explosion crater.

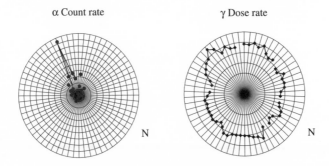

Fig. 3.12 Radiation directional distribution around the crater. (a) α counts and (b) γ dose rate.

Air in this area was also polluted by α emitters showing a level of about 10 cpm at 1 m above the ground on a windy day. The area is currently open to coal mining and land is used as pasture. Therefore, some countermeasures may be needed for protection from radiation since this former test site has been opend to access by the general population.

Fieldwork since 1995 showed negligibly small radiation risk outside but some risk remained inside the Polygon. γ-Ray dose rates in the settlements were normal with levels of less than 0.1 μSv/h. Residents currently suffer an annual dose of less than 1 mSv by the residual radioactivity from the nuclear tests. This is after suffering severe doses by the radioactive fallout in the past. High dose rates of more than 20 µSv/h were detected at several ground zero sites in the Polygon. Nuclear hazards are localized within the SNTS in the beginning of the 21st century (Fig. 3.13).

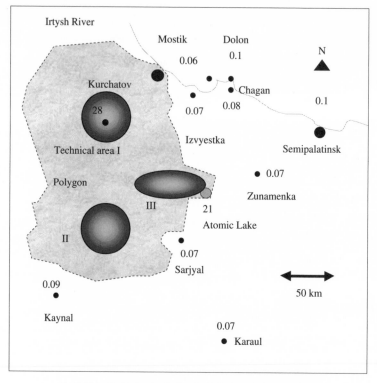

Fig. 3.13 γ Radiation in the Semipalatinsk region (after 1995).

3.6 Summary

A total of 459 nuclear tests conducted at the Semipalatinsk nuclear test site caused nuclear pollution inside the test field and radiation exposure to the population. The Kazakhstan population was exposed to radiation without being provided any official information regarding nuclear weapons tests.

The Hiroshima dosimetry team recognized external radiation exposure of up to several hundred millisieverts for residents around the test site by thermoluminescence study on brick samples. Moreover, there is no doubt that the population suffered internal exposure as well. We want to emphasize here that this dose evaluation study did not use any military data whatsoever. The technique employed was identical with the γ-ray dosimetry of the Hiroshima nuclear bomb.

Another valuable investigation result was that the present environment risk was quite low from the radiation protection point of view. The spatial dose rate was equal to or less than 0.1 micro Sv/h everywhere outside the test site. No remarkable high residual radioactivity has been observed in residential areas.

Our investigation confirmed that radioactive contamination is localized at ground zero of surface nuclear explosions inside the test site. The ground surface still showed high levels of radiation of up to 50 micro-Sv/h. Some crater explosion sites were highly contaminated by α emitters of up to 1,800 counts per minute on the surface, indicating a probable plutonium level of 1 MBq/m^2. Some countermeasures may be needed for the protection of ordinary visitors from radiation.

REFERENCES

1. J. Takada, M. Hoshi, R.I. Rozenson, S. Endo, M. Yamamoto, T. Nagatomo, T. Imanaka, B.I. Gusev, K.N. Apsalikov, N.J. Tachaijunusova, *Health Phys.*, **73**, 524 (1997)
2. J. Takada, M. Hoshi, T. Nagatomo, M. Yamamoto, S. Endo, T. Takatsuji, I. Yoshikawa, B. I. Gusev, A. Sakerbaev, N. J. Tchaijunusova, *J. Radiat. Res.*, **40**, 337 (1999)
3. The Ministry of the Russian Federation for Atomic Energy and the Ministry of Defense of the Russian Federation, *USSR Nuclear Weapons Tests and Peaceful Nuclear Explosions 1949 through 1990*, Russian Federal Nuclear Center-VNIIEF (1996)
4. U.V. Dubasov, S.A. Zelentsov, G.A. Krasilov, V.A. Logachev, A.M. Matushenko, S.G. Smagulov, B.S. Tsaturov, G.A. Tsirkov, A.K. Chernishev, *Chronological List of the Atmospheric Nuclear Tests at the Semipalatinsk Test Site and Its Radiological Characteristics*, Review of the scientific program "Semipalatinskii Poligon-Altai" **14**: 78-86 (1994) (in Russian)
5. B.I. Gusev, *Medical and Demographical Consequences of Nuclear Fallout in Some Rural Districts in the Semipalatinsk Region*, Doctoral dissertation, Almati (1993) (in Russian)
6. A.H. Tsyb, V.F. Stepanenko, V.A. Pitkevich, E.A. Ispenkov, A.V. Sevankaev, M.Y. Orlov, E.V. Dmitriev, I.A. Sapapultsev, T.L. Zhigareva, O.N. Prokofev, O.L. Obukhova, V.A. Rezontov, A.M. Matushenko, A.E. Katkov, V.N. Vyalykh, S.O. Smagulov, N. A. Meshkov, A.A. Saleev, S.E. Vidanov, *Radiologiya Meditsinskaya*, **35**(12), 1 (1990) (in Russian)
7. B.I. Gusev, *Tumor Incidence Among Inhabitants of Some Districts in the Semipalatinsk Region Exposed after Nuclear Testing at the Test Ground*, Proc. of the *2nd Hiroshima International Symposium, Hiroshima*, 153-194 (1996)
8. Y. Ichikawa, T. Higashimura, T. Sidei, *Health Phys.*, **12**, 395 (1966)
9. Y. Ichikawa, T. Nagatomo, M. Hoshi, S. Kondo, *Health Phys.*, **52**, 443 (1987)
10. W.C. Roesch, ed., *US-Japan Joint Reassessment of Atomic Bomb Radiation Dosimetry in Hiroshima and Nagasaki, Final Report*, vol.1, Radiation Effect Research Foundation, Hiroshima (1987)
11. M. J. Aitken, *Thermoluminescence Dating*, Academic Press, London (1985)
12. E. Haskell, I.K. Bailiff, *Radiat. Prot. Dosim.*, **34**, 195 (1990)
13. D. Stoneham, I.K. Bailiff, L. Brodski, H.Y. Goksu, E. Haskell, G. Hutt, H. Jungner, T. Nagatomo, *Nucl. Tracks Radiat. Meas.*, **21**, 195 (1993)

14. T. Nagatomo, M. Hoshi, Y. Ichikawa, *J. Radiat. Res.*, **33**, 211 (1992)

15 I.K. Bailiff, *Aspects of Retrospective Dosimetry Using Luminescence Techniques in Areas Contaminated by Chernobyl Fallout, Proceedings of the 2nd Hiroshima Intern. Symp.*, pp. 237-249, Res. Inst. Radiat. Biol. Med., Hiroshima Univ., Hiroshima (1999)

16. T. Imanaka, *Private Memorandum on External Doses from Fission Products on Contaminated Land after Nuclear Explosion* (1988)

17. *ICRP Publication 38*, Pergamon Press, Oxford (1983)

18. *Kazakhstan Republic (1964) Iso-dose Map.*, pp. 13-43, M-43 SSSR (in Russian)

19. J. Takada, M. Hoshi, S. Endo, V.F. Stepanenko, A.E. Kondrashov, V. Skvortsov, A. Iwanikov, D. Tikonov, Y. Gavrilin, V.P. Snykov, *Appl. Radiat. Isotopes*, **52**, 1165 (2000)

20. V.A. Logachev, *Dosimetry Map of the Semipalatinsk Region, Fixative Exposure Iso-dose of the Very Dangerous Nuclear Explosions* (I-XXI) (1949-1965) (1965) (in Russian)

21. J. Takada, V.E. Stepanov, D.P. Yefremov, T. Shintani, A. Akiyama, M. Fukuda, M. Hoshi, *J. Radiat. Res.*, **40**, 223 (1999)

22. US Department of Defense and the Energy Research and Development Administration, *The Effects of Nuclear Weapons*, U.S. Government Printing Office, Washington D.C. (1977)

23. V.M. Loborev, Y.N. Shoikhet, V.V. Sudakov, V.I. Zelenov, M.N. Gabbasov, *Doses of Residents of the Cities of Semipalatinsk, Ust-Kamenogorsk, Kurchatov and the Settlement of Chagan Delivered by the Nuclear Tests at the Semipalatinsk Test Site*, Scientific Preprogram "Semipalatinsk Poligon-Altai" **1** (13), 51-64 (1997)

4

Toward Resettlement on Rongelap Island

The nuclear disaster which remains unforgotten in the mind of the Japanese people following Hiroshima and Nagasaki is the thermonuclear test explosion that was unleashed on Bikini Atoll by the United States in 1954. In July 1999, the author had the opportunity to investigate Rongelap Atoll where the population had suffered hazardous fallout from the Bikini explosion. The inhabitants were told by the U.S. that their island was safe and they returned to Rongelap in 1957. However, in 1985 they feared radiological pollution and left the island of their own will. This chapter is a report consisting mainly of local investigation results.

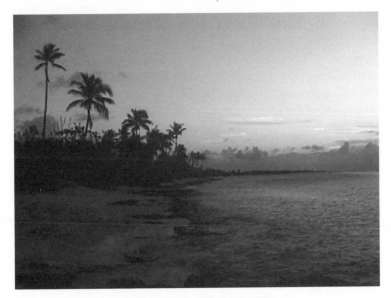

Fig. 4.1 Rongelap Island, July 1999.

4.1 A Brief History of the Nuclear Disaster on Rongelap Island

The U.S.A. began nuclear weapons tests in the Marshall Islands in the Pacific Ocean in 1946, the year follwing the end of the Pacific War. Sixty-five tests with a

TNT equivalent of 108 Mt were conducted on the Bikini Atoll and in the northern part of Enowetok Atoll until 1958.[1]

The biggest nuclear explosion was the BRAVO test of a thermonuclear weapon with an output of 15 Mt that occurred on Bikini at 6:45 on March 1, 1954. This explosive power is 1,000 times that of the Hiroshima nuclear bomb and is equal nearly to the 18 Mt total output for the 459 nuclear weapons tests conducted in the Semipalatinsk region. A Japanese fishing boat, the *Fukuryumaru No.5*, was exposed to fallout from this explosion, as were the residents in the northeastern parts of Rongelap, Rongeric and Utrik atolls, where fallout was carried by the wind.

Fallout began on Rongelap Atoll 175 km from Bikini about four hours after the explosion. Radioactive white coral powder accumulated with a thickness of 2–3 cm. Sixty-four islanders were rescued by the U.S. Army at 10:00 on March 3, 51 hours later.[2] Also, 18 islanders who were staying on Sifo Island of Ailinginae Atoll were rescued 54 hours later. Whole-body dose of radiation was estimated to be 1.9 Gy and 1.1 Gy for the former and latter, respectively. Acute dermatitis, heaving, diarrhea and other symptoms occurred until rescue. Hair started falling out after the rescued islanders arrived at the Kwajalein U.S. Army Base.

The *Fukuryumaru No.5* was fishing on the northern side of the Rongelap Atoll, about 150 km from the epicenter. The crews witnessed the flash of BRAVO. Three hours after the explosion, fallout reached the boat. The radioactivity of the material which piled up on the deck was estimated to be 26 GBq/m.[2,3]

The return of the islanders to their home atoll of Rongelap was approved by the Atomic Energy Commission in March 1957. Two hundred fifty islanders returned to Rongelap Island on June 29. The dose rate there was 0.26 μGy/h.[3]

The Department of Energy (DOE) investigated the radiation condition on all 11 atolls. The results were published in the Marshall language in 1982. The

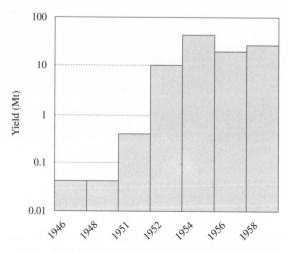

Fig. 4.2 USA nuclear weapons tests on the Marshall Islands.[4]

contents of this report became a cause of fear for the Rongelap people, and the islanders expressed their desire to immigrate to Washington and the Marshall Island government. They were refused, so the islanders left the island on their own with the cooperation of Greenpeace, the international environmental protection group. In May 1985, the islanders boarded a large sailboat, the *Rainbow Warrior*, and started to live on Mejatto Island of Kwajalein Atoll.[3]

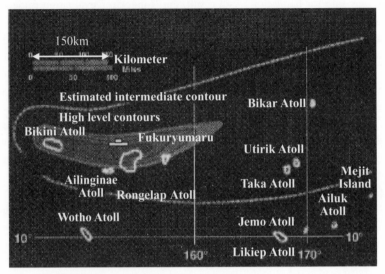

Fig. 4.3 Fallout pattern of the Bravo explosion in 1954.
[Reproduced with permission from W.L. Robison, C. Sun, *Health Phys.*, **73**, 152 (1997)]

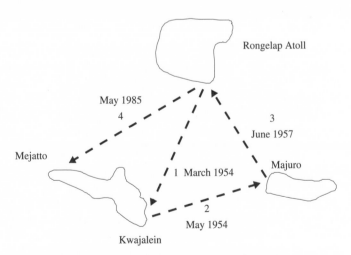

Fig. 4.4 The movement of the Rongelap people since 1954.
[Reproduced with permission from L.C. Sun, J.H. Clinton, E. Kaplan, C.B. Meinhold, *Health Phys.*, **73**, 86 (1997)]

4.2 Resettlement Program of Rongelap Island[5]

In August 1987, the Republic of the Marshall Islands requested Dr. Henry Kohn, former chairperson of the Bikini Reconstruction Committee, to chair a review of the 1982 DOE Report.[3] The purpose of the review was to judge whether Rongelap Island was safe for habitation. As a result, the Rongelap reevaluation project was started.

The committee issued a report in July 1988 stating that Rongelap's main island was generally safe for life, if the inhabitants ate meals comprising a mix of food produced locally and imported food. However, the report states that the radioactive dose for infants and small children is another potential cause of concern.

A Memorandum of Understanding (MOU) was signed by the Republic of the Marshall Islands, the Rongelap Atoll district government, the U.S. Department of Energy and the U.S. Department of the Interior in 1992. Two independent investigations were conducted by Rongelap and the DOE as a result.

Conditions of Resettlement in the Southern Area of Rongelap Atoll
(1) If the maximally exposed persons living on Rongelap Island and eating only locally produced food showed levels exceeding 1mSv/y, and
(2) if soil concentrations of transuranics on Rongelap Island exceeded 7.4 kBq/m^2.

As part of this agreement, the U.S. Department of the Interior paid the Rongelap Local Government US\$ 1.6 million to fund scientific investigations and for living expenses. The Rongelap Local Government subsequently established the Rongelap Resettlement Project and contracted a scientific management team to evaluate the expected radiation dose of the returning population.

In January 1991, the Marshall Islands Nationwide Radiological Study, supported by the Marshall Islands Government, completed the construction of a dedicated radiological laboratory in Majuro, the capital city of the Marshall Islands. This scientific project was based on P.L. 99–239 of the Compact of Free Association signed by President Ronald Reagan in 1986. For five years (1990-1994), the Marshall Islands Government implemented an independent program, evaluating radiation conditions on 29 atolls. This was the first systematic investigation conducted on all the atolls.

Most of the monitoring was done by *in-situ* γ-ray spectrometry on more than 400 islands. The samples included tropical fruits such as coconuts, over 200 soil depth profiles and over 800 surface soil samples. They were examined for concentration of cesium-137 (Cs-137) and all the other γ-ray emitters. Surface soil was also analyzed for plutonium-239, -240 (Pu-239, -240). S.L. Simon and J. Graham were in charge of these studies.[1]

Four independent dose assessments were reported in 1994, and it was concluded that there was a possibility that 25 percent of the adult population had a dose of over 1 mSv/y when living on Rongelap Island and taking in only local food.[14]

In September 1996, the Clinton Administration announced a donation of US$ 45 million for the Rongelap Islanders Resettlement Plan. Phase 1 of Rongelap Island in Rongelap Atoll was established in January 1998. Construction of the necessary infrastructure and partial clean-up in some areas was initiated based on this plan.

4.3 Radiation Survey of Rongelap Atoll in 1999

The Resettlement Program of Rongelap Island, the main island of Rongelap Atoll of the Marshall Islands started in July 1998.[5] Radiological investigation and the information obtained is of great importance for the people of Rongelap. A survey of Rongelap Island in the atoll was begun in 1999 in collaboration with the Bumbum Project.[6,7] The author and his team arrived on Rongelap Island on July 6 on the fishing boat, the *Riemannman*.

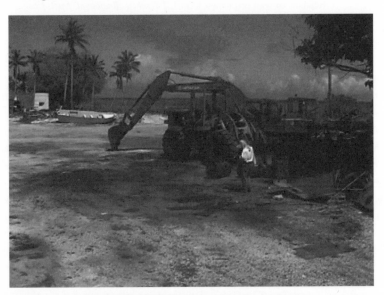

Fig. 4.5 Construction on Rongelap Island in 1999.

Radiation surveys, *in-situ* spectroscopy and soil sampling for plutonium analysis were carried out. Portable whole-body counting of Cs-137 was also carried out on workers of Rongelap Island who may take in radioactivity by food or inhalation.

We investigated 17 sites covering the entire area of Rongelap Island, which is about 8 km long and 0.2–1 km wide, as shown in Fig. 4.6. The γ-ray dose rate (1 cm dose equivalent rate) was measured in the present study using a pocket survey meter (Aloka PDR-101) in which a CsI (Tl) (20 × 25 × 15 mm) detector is installed.

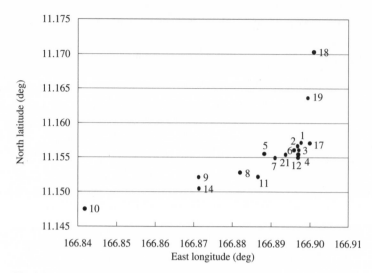

Fig. 4.6 A map of the radiation survey sites on Rongelap Island.
[Reproduced with permission from J. Takada, *J. Radioanal. Nucl. Chem.*, **252**, 262 (2002) ©Kluwer Academic Publishers]

Core soil was sampled for plutonium analysis using a stainless steel pipe with an inner diameter of 47 mm to a depth of about 300 mm. Determination of plutonium isotopes was conducted by radiochemical separation. Activity of Pu-239, -240 was measured by α-ray spectroscopy. The details of this procedure have been described elsewhere.[8]

Abnormal radiological value was not observed at all 17 sites including the beach we investigated on Rongelap Island, as shown in Table 4.1. The residual radioactivity on the island was quite low in 1999. Indeed, the maximum Cs-137 contamination was 39 kBq/m². This value, which is ten times higher than values in Japan due to the global fallout of world wide nuclear tests, is much lower than the values in areas highly contaminated due to the Chernobyl accident.[9,10] The value in Zaborie village, the most contaminated area in Russia due to the Chernobyl accident, was 6.3 MBq/m² maximum in 1997.[9] The maximum α and β count rates in surface soil were 1 cpm and 182 cpm, respectively, no higher than the values in the Hiroshima bay area.

The maximum value (0.033 μSv/h) of γ-ray dose rate on Rongelap Island was lower than values (~ 0.1 μSv/h) in radiologically clean areas of Japan and resident areas near the Semipalatinsk nuclear test site.[10] The mean annual external dose for whole-body due to Cs-137 was estimated to be 0.096 mSv/y where the natural background dose rate was assumed to be 0.012 μSv/h, as shown in Fig. 4.7.

We found relatively low radiation and activity in the clean-up area where surface soil of up to 30 cm in depth was removed on the central island. According to the Resettlement Program of Rongelap Island in Rongelap Atoll, the surface soil will be removed for each residence.[5]

Table 4.1 Data of the radiological survey on Rongelap Island in July 1999

Site[*1]	GPS coordinates (deg)		Cs-137 (kBq/m^2)	γ Dose rate (μSv/h)	Count rate (cpm)	
	E	N			β	α
99RLI01	166.897	11.157	7.8	0.017	143	0
99RLI02	166.897	11.157	5.2	0.015	109	0
99RLI03	166.897	11.156	1.3	0.012	88	0
		Max.	7.8	0.017	143	0
		Av.	6.5	0.015	126	0
		Min.	1.3	0.012	88	0
99RLI04	166.897	11.156	22.2	0.024	111	0
99RLI05	166.888	11.155	30.1	0.025	120	0
99RLI06	166.897	11.155	21.3	0.028	127	1
99RLI07	166.891	11.155	32.2	0.030	182	1
99RLI08	166.882	11.153	32.8	0.027	134	1
99RLI09	166.871	11.152	39.3	0.033	128	1
99RLI10	166.841	11.147	2.08	0.010	83	0
99RLI11	166.887	11.152	nm[*2]	nm	90	1
99RLI12	166.896	11.156	nm	nm	72	nm
99RLI14	166.871	11.150	nm	nm	85	nm
99RLI17	166.900	11.157	nm	nm	69	nm
99RLI18	166.901	11.170	nm	nm	88	nm
99RLI19	166.900	11.164	29.6	0.031	114	0
99RLI21	166.894	11.155	21.8	0.024	133	nm
		Max.	39.3	0.033	182	1
		Av.	25.7	0.026	110	0.56
		Min.	2.1	0.010	69	0

[*1] Sites 99RLI01-3 were in the clean-up area.

[*2] nm = not measured.

Cs-137: one measurement at one site

γ Dose rate, β count rate: average value of data taken at each corner of triangle with sides 5 m long.

α Count rate: maximum value of data taken at each corner of triangle with sides 5 m long.

α, β Count rate: active area is 72 cm^2 for the counting

[Reproduced with permission from J. Takada, *J. Radioanal. Nucl. Chem.*, **252**, 263 (2002) ©Kluwer Academic Publishers]

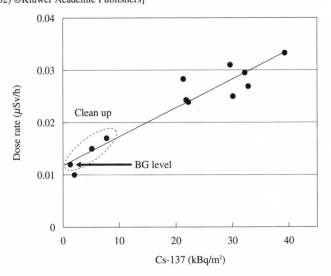

Fig. 4.7 Radiation conditions (γ dose rate and Cs-137 contaminations) on Rongelap Island in 1999.
[Reproduced with permission from J. Takada, *J. Radioanal. Nucl. Chem.*, **252**, 263 (2002) ©Kluwer Academic Publishers]

Activity of Pu-239, 240 at two sites on Rongelap Island was found to be 3.1 and 3.6 kBq/m² respectively. More than 90% of the activity of plutonium was kept at a depth of between 0 and 10 cm under the surface of the ground, as shown in Table 4.3.

4.3.1 Cesium-137 Body Burden in Workers

One important measurement is the whole-body count of Cs-137 as well as environment investigation on the island. This makes internal dose evaluation possible. A survey on Rongelap islanders was carried out by the Brookhaven National Laboratory between 1977 and 1984.

Although food for workers was imported, some of them often eat local food such as pork, chicken, fish and tropical fruits on Rongelap Island. Such intake of local food may not have exceeded 10 %. Moreover, they are exposed to radionuclides through inhalation during construction of roads, airports and soil clean-up. The results were given to each person by a document in the Marshall language just after the examination. The body burden of Cs-137 in six of 15 workers was not a value to raise anxiety as far as internal exposure was concerned.

The whole-body count of Cs-137 for these six workers indicated a mean value of 27 ± 11 Bq/kg (2.0 ± 0.7 kBq). This value is three orders of magnitude less than the annual limit of intake of Cs-137 according to ICRP Publication 30 on occupational exposure.[11] The internal dose rate can be estimated by the following equation,[12]

Internal effective dose rate (mS/y) =
$2.55 \times 1.4 \times 10^{-2}$ (mSv/kBq) × Body content (kBq)   (4.1)

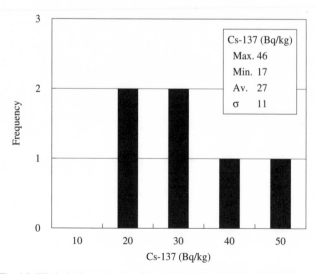

Fig. 4.8 Whole-body count of workers on Rongelap Island in July 1999.
[Reproduced with permission from J. Takada, *J. Radioanal. Nucl. Chem.*, **252**, 264 (2002) ©Kluwer Academic Publishers]

The annual internal dose was estimated to be 0.07 ± 0.03 mSv/y for workers on Rongelap Island in 1999. This value is less than the 0.26 ± 0.08 mSv/y which was calculated from data of whole-body measurements for Rongelap people between 1977 and 1984 by the Brookhaven National Laboratory.[13] Therefore the internal dose appears to be decreasing with decrease in environmental radioactivity.

4.4 Recovery from Nuclear Hazard on Rongelap Island and Islands to the North

The areas on Rongelap Island severely contaminated by radiological fallout in 1954 have been recovering year by year, as shown in Fig. 4.9. The data for land contamination in 1974 and 1994 and for human body between 1977 and 1984 are taken from Walker (1997),[14] Simon (1997)[15] and Robinson (1997),[13] respectively. The decrease in effective half-life of Cs-137 in the ground, which is estimated to be 6.6 y, is much shorter than the physical half-life of Cs-137 (30 y).

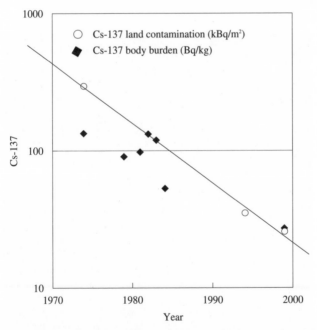

Fig. 4.9 Cs-137 in the land and inhabitants of Rongelap Island as a function of time. [Reproduced with permission from J. Takada, *J. Radioanal. Nucl. Chem.*, **252**, 264 (2002) ©Kluwer Academic Publishers]

This causes decrease in the body burden of Cs-137, as shown in the same figure. The radioactivitiy on a coral island whose sea level is only 1.5–2.0 m may have been swept away by the large waves of the Pacific Ocean. The effective transfer constant [ratio between body burden (kBq/kg) and land contamination (kBq/m²)] of Cs-137 is estimated to be 0.77 ± 0.33 (10^{-3}m²/kg) on Rongelap Island using the data set and fitting function of Fig. 4.9. This effective factor between human and environment includes not only natural components but social components as well. The case of Rongelap Island involves factors such as imported food and food from northern islands, which was more contaminated by radioactivity.

Total effective dose, which was estimated to be 0.17 mSv/y due to Cs-137 for residents in the Rongelap Island 1999 study, is much less than the 1 mSv/y dose limit for public exposure recommended in 1990 by the International Commission on Radiological Protection.[16]

We noted that activity of Pu-239, -240 in soil (80 Bq/kg in the top 5 cm and 3.4 kBq/m^2 at two sites) in the Rongelap Island 1999 project was lower than previous values. The activities for soil sampled in 1978[13] and around 1994[15] were 117 and 133 Bq/kg, respectively. Plutonium may decrease more slowly than Cs-137 in the environment.

Radiological information for the entire atoll will be needed for the people of Rongelap after their return to their home island, since most of the farms producing local food are located on the northern islands. We investigated Kaballe and

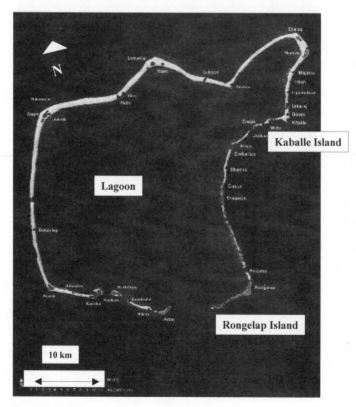

Fig. 4.10 Field investigation map of Rongelap Atoll.
[From *The Meaning of Radiation for those Atolls in the Northern Parts of the Marshall Islands that Were Surveyed in 1978*, Department of Energy, USA (1982)]

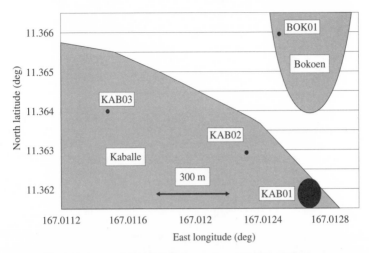

Fig. 4.11 A map of the radiation survey sites on Kaballe and Bokoen.

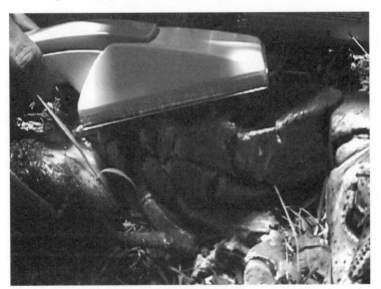

Fig. 4.12 Coconut crab on Kaballe.

Table 4.2 Data of the radiological survey on Kaballe and Bokoen islands in July 1999

Site	GPS coordinates (deg)		Cs-137 (kBq/m²)	γ Dose rate (μSv/h)	Count rate (cpm)	
	E	N			β	α
99KAB01	167.0127	11.362	3400	0.727	1205	2
99KAB02	167.0123	11.363	96.5	0.064	247	1
99KAB03	167.0115	11.364	120	0.074	211	2
99BOK01	167.0125	11.366	3.2	0.007	255	0

Cs-137: one measurement at one site
γ Dose rate, β count rate: average value of data taken at each corner of triangle with sides 5 m long
α Count rate: maximum value of data taken at each corner of triangle with sides 5 m long
α, β Count rate: active area is 72 cm² for the counting
[Reproduced with permission from J. Takada, *J. Radioanal. Nucl. Chem.*, **252**, 263 (2002) ©Kluwer Academic Publishers]

Table 4.3 Concentration of Pu-239, -240 in soil samples
from Rongelap (RLC) and Kaballe (KBC)
islands.

Sample number	Depth (cm)	Pu-239, -240 concentration		
		(Bq/kg)		(Bq/m²)
RLC21-0	0-5	71.37	± 2.99	1889.1
RLC21-5	5-10	26.58	± 0.83	1035.6
RLC21-10	10-15	4.36	± 0.23	143.2
RLC21-15	15-20	0.58	± 0.04	16.1
RLC21-20	20-27	0.16	± 0.02	9.9
	Total			3093.9
RLC4-0	0-5	87.98	± 2.19	2292.4
RLC4-5	5-10	36.44	± 1.26	1045.2
RLC4-10	10-15	3.68	± 0.21	110.8
RLC4-15	15-20	2.12	± 0.11	99.0
RLC4-20	20-30	1.55	± 0.09	102.5
	Total			3649.9
KBC3-0	0-5	293.50	± 16.36	11108.3
KBC3-5	5-10	114.88	± 6.87	3978.9
KBC3-10	10-15	15.55	± 0.55	697.8
KBC3-15	15-22	8.73	± 0.35	698.8
	Total			16483.8

[Reproduced with permission from J. Takada, *J. Radioanal. Nucl. Chem.*, **252**, 265 (2002) ©Kluwer Academic Publishers]

Bokoen Islands, which are located 25 km northeast of Rongelap Island. Radioactive contamination on Kaballe was still high in 1999. We found that one site near a beach was highly contaminated with maximum levels of Cs-137 of 3.4 MBq/m², α-rays of 2 cpm, β-rays of 1205 cpm and γ-rays of 0.73 μSv/h. Activity of Pu-239, -240 in soil at one site was 294 Bq/kg (top 5 cm) and 16.5 kBq/m².

4.5 Summary

Rongelap Island was polluted by fallout from a thermonuclear explosion of 15 Mt in 1954. If the islanders had not been evacuated from the island, all would have died.

A small island with a sea level of only 2 m is washed by the waves of the Pacific Ocean. After the Bikini Atoll nuclear disaster, nuclear pollution on Rongelap decreased with an effective half-life of seven years. Surface radioactivity, which was probably several GBq/m² at the time of the disaster, decreased to 1/100,000 45 years later. The environment, which indicated 28 mSv/h on the day following the explosion, recovered to 0.02 μSv/h in 45 years.

In 1957 there may still have existed radiation exposure which could not be ignored on Rongelap Island due to residual radioactivity. The islanders, who were very concerned, left the island in 1985 and began to live on another small island. A resettlement program was started in 1998.

The results of the investigation conducted in July 1999 were summarized and sent to the people of Rongelap in October 2000. The results showed substantial recovery of the environment and proved to be good news for the islanders. The problem of the islands north of Rongelap Atoll remains uninvestigated, but the radiation risk to life on Rongelap Island is quite small.

REFERENCES

1. S.L. Simon, J.C. Graham. *Findings of the Nationwide Radiological Study, Summary Report*, Republic of the Marshall Islands, Majuro (1994)
2. E.P. Cronkite, R.A. Conard, V.P. Bond, *Health Phys.*, **73**, 176 (1997)
3. S.L. Simon, *Health Phys.*, **73**, 5 (1997)
4. B.B. Bennett, L.E. DE Deer, A. Doury, in: *Nuclear Weapons Test Programs of Different Countries, Nuclear Test Explosions* (F. Warner, R.J.C. Kirchmann, eds.), SCOPE59, p.13, John Wiley and Sons, Chichester (2000)
5. *Rongelap Atoll Resettlement Plan Phase I*, Rongelap Atoll Local Government Rongelap Local Distribution Authority (1998)
6. Bumbum Project, *A Non-governmental Organization for Helping the Local Society of Rongelap People*, was established in 1996. http://www.erix.com/bumbum/
7. J. Takada, *J. Radioanal. Nucl. Chem.*, **252**, 262 (2002)
8. M. Yamamoto, M. Hoshi, J. Takada, A. Kh. Sakerbaev, B.I. Gusev, *J. Radioanal. Nucl. Chem.*, **242**, 63 (1999)
9. J. Takada, M. Hoshi, S. Endo, V.F. Stepanenko, A.E. Kondrashov, D. Petin, V. Skvortsov, A. Ivannikov, D. Tikounov, Y. Gavrilin, V.P. Snykov, *Applied Radiation and Isotopes*, **52**, 1165 (2000)
10. J. Takada, M. Hoshi, R.I. Rozenson, S. Endo, M. Yamamoto, T. Nagatomo, T. Imanaka, B.I. Gusev, K.N. Apsalikov, N.J. Tachaijunusova, *Health Phys.*, **73**, 524 (1997)
11. *ICRP Publication 30, Part 1, Limits of Intakes of Radionuclides by Workers*, Pergamon Press, Oxford (1978)
12. L.C. Sun, J.H. Clinton, E. Kaplan, C.B. Meinhold, *Health Phys.*, **73**, 86 (1997)
13. W.L. Robison, C. Sun, *Health Phys.*, **73**, 152 (1997)
14. R.B. Walker, S. P. Gessel, E.E. Held, *Health Phys.*, **73**, 223 (1997)
15. S.L. Simon, W.L. Robinson, M.C. Thorne, L.H. Toburen, B. Franke, K.F. Baverstock, H.J. Pettingill, *Health Phys.*, **73**, 133 (1997)
16. *ICRP Publication 60, 1990 Recommendations of the International Commission on Radiological Protection*, Pergamon Press, Oxford (1991)

5

Nuclear Explosions Conducted for Peaceful Purposes

After 1963, when the Limited Test Ban Treaty went into effect, nuclear explosions were implemented near the surface of the earth for "peaceful purposes" by the USA and the USSR.[1] These nuclear explosions caused great amounts of nuclear pollution on the earth's surface in addition to releasing much radioactive material into the atmosphere. Approximately 100 "peaceful nuclear explosions" were conducted by the two countries. Between 1962 and 1968, six nuclear explosions of this type were conducted in Nevada, U.S.A. The largest of these was a 104-kt explosion in 1962, which formed a crater. The second largest explosion was one of 30 kt in 1968. The others were explosions of less than 10 kt. In this chapter, we review the nuclear explosions for industrial purposes conducted in the former USSR.

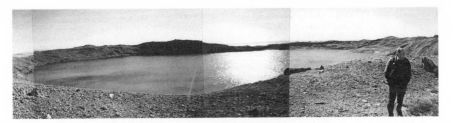

Fig. 5.1 Atomic Lake at the Semipalatinsk Test Site.

5.1 Industrial Application of Nuclear Explosions in the Former USSR

The former Soviet Union conducted 124 nuclear explosions for the industrial purposes of stratum investigation, earthwork at dams and waste storage facilities, the production of natural gas and petroleum in the period 1965-1988.[2] Most were explosions on a scale of 2 to 20 kt at a depth of 500–2000 m. However, some of them should be classified as surface explosions. They occurred after the Limited Test Ban Treaty had already been signed.

Underground nuclear explosions are physically classified into three kinds: effective explosions on the surface of the earth, shallow underground explosions and explosions at sufficient depth. According to this order, such explosions become hazardous for environmental pollution and area residents being exposed to radiation. Since the fireball goes out of the ground in shallow explosions, this type should be physically classified as a surface nuclear explosion. The epicenter is polluted by fission products, neutron-induced radioactivity and plutonium. This is the worst type of nuclear explosion. In this case, inhabitants living downwind are exposed to radioactive cloud. Since radioactive gas escapes from cracks in the ground in a relatively shallow explosion, safety cannot be assured.

On the other hand, since radioactive material is stored underground in explosions of sufficient depth, they are comparatively safe. However, there is concern that pollution will spread in the basin system and to the surface of the earth via underground water which flows through numerous cracks.

In the case of underground explosions near the surface of the earth, ground material of considerable quantity evaporates at very high temperatures. This is sucked up by the updraft which occurs when the fireball rises. Then, by the rapid expansion of the high-pressure and high-temperature gases from the point of explosion, rocks on the surface of the earth are moved and a crater forms. Such a crater consists of the following three layers: the top layer formed by the material that accumulates after having been blown up into the air, the second layer which

Table 5.1 Industrial nuclear explosions in Russia

Purpose	Number of times
Seismological research	33
Oil and gas extraction	21
Underground reservoirs for oil and gas	19
Underground reservoirs for toxic liquid wastes	2
Sealing natural gas well	1
Miscellaneous	5
Total	81

[Reproduced with permission from V. Larin, E. Tar, *Bulletin of the Atomic Scientists*, May/June, 19 (1999)]

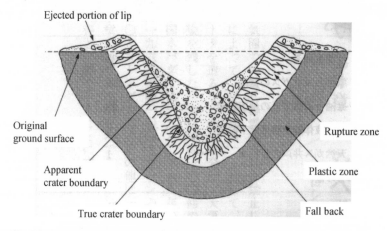

Fig. 5.2 Cross-sectional view of crater formed by nuclear explosion.
[From US Department of Defense, *The Effects of Nuclear Weapons* (1977)]

has countless cracks and the third layer which has been permanently transformed by the explosion.[3] The radius of the second crack layer is about 1.5 times the radius of the crater.

5.2 Dam Construction Involving Nuclear Explosion

The first industrial application of a nuclear explosion in the USSR was implemented in the Barapan area of the Semipalatinsk nuclear test site on January 15, 1965.[5] A thermonuclear bomb of 140 kt output exploded at a depth of 175 m near the east boundary of the test site. This output corresponds to a fireball radius of 400 m in the case of an air explosion. A crater of about 400 m diameter and 100 m deep was formed. After the explosion, many workers were forced to engage in the construction of a reservoir around the crater. This is now called Atomic Lake (Fig. 5.1).

At the time of the first investigation conducted by the author and his team in 1995,[6] the dose rate was 10 μSv/h, which was more than 100 times that of the natural background, i.e., the crater surface of considerable thickness was polluted by radioactive material resulting from nuclear fission products and neutron capture.

Although this was claimed to be a nuclear explosion for a peaceful purpose, it

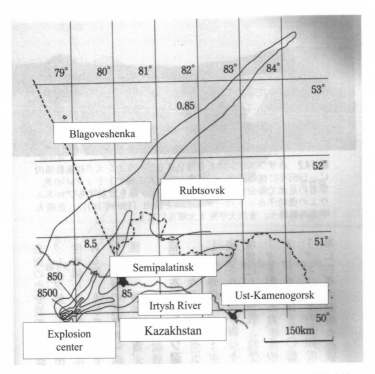

Fig. 5.3 Isodose rate map following the 140-kt nuclear explosion of January 15, 1965, 24 hours after. [Reproduced with permission from J. Takada, *Nuclear Test Explosions, SCOPE59,* ©John Wiley & Sons (2000)]

was a dangerous and reckless event. Nuclear explosion is not suited to earthwork because of the nuclear pollution which remains.

A great deal of radioactive material from this explosion was spread in a dust pillar 2,500 m high, according to Dr. Youri Israel of the Institute of Global Climate and Ecology in Moscow.[4] The pillar moved in the northeastern direction toward Semipalatinsk City as it spread. In this way, earth dust with huge radioactivity released from the nuclear explosion polluted the environment downwind from the site of explosion and exposed inhabitants of the area to radiation. Radiation in Semipalatinsk City 24 hours after the explosion was recorded to be 8.5 μSv/h.

At 3–4 hours after the explosion, the radiation can be 10 times higher than the above level. The village of Zunamenka is located approximately midway between Semipalatinsk City and the point of explosion. The author assumes the radiation in the village as being 1 mSv/h at H + 3–4.

5.3 Underground Nuclear Explosions in Sakha

The Sakha region is rich in underground resources such as diamond, gold, silver, tungsten, ironstone, coal, petroleum and natural gas. Its diamond production comprises 20% of the annual world output. There is a crater of 4 km diameter and 500 m deep at the diamond mine in Mirnny.

Twelve underground nuclear explosions (UNEs) with industrial applications were conducted in the Sakha region of the Russian Federation between 1974 and 1987. Fig. 5.4 shows a schematic time-table of the UNEs with information of output in kilotons and underground depth, taken from Yakimets (1996).[7] Most of the UNEs were carried out at a depth of 500 to 1500 m. The maximum yield was 20 kt. Four UNEs were conducted for a geological study of deep seismic waves of the Earth's crust, six UNEs to intensify oil recovery and gas inflow, one UNE to obtain underground crude oil and one UNE (named Crystal) for the building of a dam for the storage of waste after the extraction of useful components from ore.

The environmental radiation was of natural background level at 10 nuclear explosion sites according to a report of the Ministry of Atomic Energy of Russian Federation. However, two UNEs, Crystal (2 kt, –100 m, 1974) and Kraton-3 (20 kt, –525 m, 1978) failed with radioactive releases to the environment. In Crystal in 1974, an area of a radius of 60 m showed high levels of pollution. The government implemented countermeasures. A sanitary zone with a rocky embankment 15 m high and 150 m in diameter was formed over the explosion site of Crystal in 1992.[8] Kraton-3 was conducted in an effort to produce an artificial earthquake wave in 1978 but ended in failure. A seal was blown off, allowing nuclear fission products to escape and be spread by the wind. The external dose along the pathway of the radioactive cloud was estimated to be 5,000–250 mGy at locations between 3 and 13 km from the explosion site. The average individual dose was estimated to be 100 mSv. A forest of larch trees in the path of the radioactive cloud 3.5 km from the accident site had died by the summer in 1979. A ground

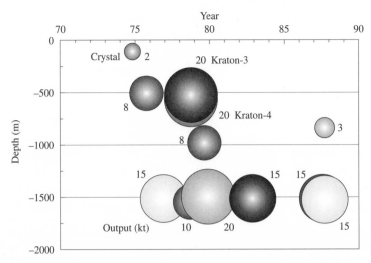

Fig. 5.4 Twelve underground nuclear explosions in Sakha from 1974 to 1987. Data of the UNEs are taken from Yakimets (1996).[7] The radius of the balloon is proportional to the output of the explosion. The radius of the balloon is proportional to the output of the explosion.
[From J. Takada et al., *J. Rad. Res.*, **40**, 224 (1999)]

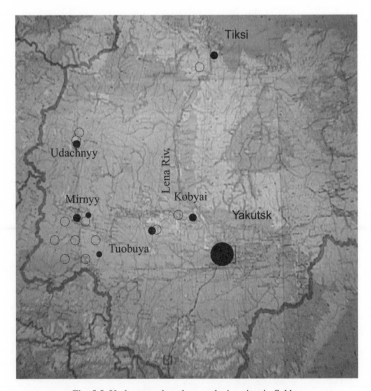

Fig. 5.5 Underground nuclear explosion sites in Sakha.

surface area of 500 m^2 at the hypocenter and the path of the radioactive cloud was cultivated to weaken the effect of the radioactivity of the plutonium-239 (Pu-239), strontium-90 (Sr-90), cesium-137 (Cs-137) and other radioactive materials in 1990. Polluted equipment and soil were buried in a trench 2.5 m deep and covered with clean soil 1 m thick. A hill 2.5 m high above the drilling hole was built using clean soil.

The Institute of Radiation Hygiene carried out field investigations on the two sites in autumn 1996 and reported severe radioactive contamination and doses.[8,9] Pollution by Pu-239, -240 of 0.3–7.5 kBq/kg, Cs-137 of 0.12–5.2 kBq/kg and Sr-90 of 0.05–0.8 kBq/kg in soil sampled at Crystal site was reported. Around Kraton-3, the maximum level of Pu-239, -240 was 4.3 kBq/kg, that of Cs-137 was 82 kBq/kg and that of Sr-90 was 99 kBq/kg. The dose rate was 50 μSv/h.

5.4 Radiological Conditions around Kraton-4

In March 1998 the author and his coworkers conducted a radiological survey (γ-survey and *in-situ* spectroscopy in the field and for local foodstuffs) of the Kraton-4 (K-4) area in response to requests from the Ministry of Nature Protection of the Sakha Republic made to Japan.[10]

The K-4 explosion with an output of 20 kt was conducted at a depth of 560 m on August 9, 1978. However, as a result of the explosion, multiple cracks in the ground surface appeared, causing three new islands to emerge in nearby Lake Nijili, and water and sand banks appeared within a radius of 500–600 m from the bare hole.[6] A rise in the water level of the lake resulted in a shoreline shift of 8-10 m.

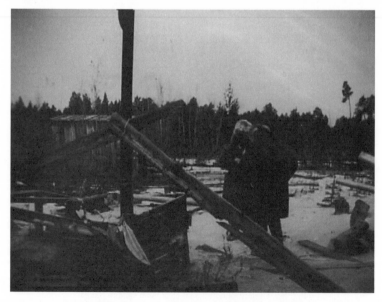

Fig. 5.6 Hypocenter of the Kraton-4 explosion of 20 kt.

Surface contamination due to a deep UNE is not well understood since nuclear test sites always include ground and atmospheric explosions resulting in radioactive contamination of the ground surface.[6,11,12] Nuclear explosions in Sakha were generally conducted underground. The K-4 site is more than 200 km from the other UNE sites, making it suitable for the study of leakage of radioactivity from the epicenter to the ground surface.

The environmental radiation dose was measured in the present study using a pocket survey meter (Aloka PDR-101) in which a CsI (Tl) (20 × 25 × 15 mm) detector was installed. The range was 0.001–19.99 μSv/h. With this meter, the environmental dose rate was measured with an error of 15%. The *in-situ* measurement of γ-ray spectra was carried out to detect Cs-137 contamination on the ground surface and in local foodstuffs using a portable NaI spectrometer (Hamamatsu C-3475) with an NaI scintillator (2.5 cmϕ × 5.1 cm) and a multichannel analyzer with 128 channels. The surface density of Cs-137 activity on the ground was calculated with a converting constant from the counting rate to surface density of Cs-137, which was calibrated to contaminated territory near Chernobyl. Moreover, a detector which had been calibrated for whole-body counting of Cs-137 was used to detect radioactivity in pieces of raw meat.

Figure 5.7 is a map of K-4 and other UNE sites together with radiation dose rates measured at 5 different places, (a) K-4 hypocenter, (b) in the middle of Lake Dukayan, which is about 4 km from the hypocenter, (c) a place on the ground 100 m from the shore of Lake Dukayan, (d) Teya village, 21 km from the hypocenter and (e) Yakutsk, 280 km from the hypocenter. The dose rate at each place is expressed as the average of those measured at 3 points within 10 m. The dose rate at the K-4 hypocenter (0.022 μSv/h) was much lower than that at Teya village, and more than 10 times lower than those at Crystal and Kraton-3 hypocenters reported by Miretsky et al.[8] The low dose rate for iced Lake Dukayan suggested

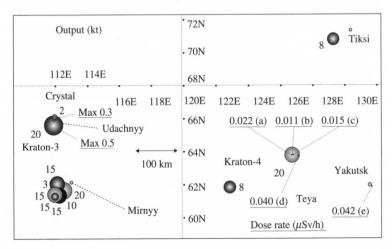

Fig. 5.7 Results of dose rate measurements made around K-4 and other sites are shown on the map with coordinates (E, N).
[From J. Takada et al., *J. Rad. Res.*, **40**, 225 (1999)]

little radioactive contamination of the water. Therefore, the dose rates at these five places as determined by the present measurements were within the normal range.

This was confirmed by measuring the environmental dose rates just around the K-4 hypocenter. Fig. 5.8 shows dose rate as a function of distance from the hypocenter of K-4. Although the ground surface was covered with snow of about 40 cm thickness, the measured dose rates were very low, ranging from 0.014 to 0.028 µSv/h. This compares with natural background values in other countries such as Japan and Kazakhstan.[6] The mean value around the hypocenter was 0.022 ± 0.004 µSv/h for 9 spots within a 1 km range. We did not observe a high level of radiation around the hypocenter.

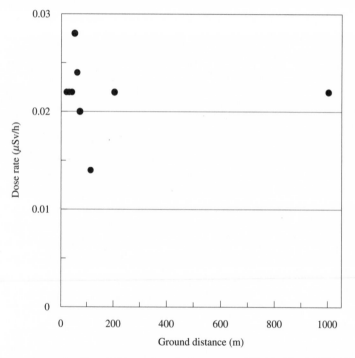

Fig. 5.8 Dose rate as a function of distance from the hypocenter of K-4 in March 1998. The ground surface was covered with snow 40 cm thick.
[From J. Takada et al., *J. Rad. Res.*, **40**, 226 (1999)]

Figure 5.9 shows the results of *in-situ* measurements of γ-ray spectra at the K-4 hypocenter, Lake Dukayan and Yakutsk. The spectrum at the K-4 hypocenter did not show any remarkable γ-ray peak from fission products such as Cs-137 with a half-life of 30 y. The effective surface contamination of Cs-137 at the hypocenter was estimated to be less than the detectable limit of 1.1 kBq/m², which is in marked contrast to that reported at the K-3 hypocenter (Cs-137: 82 kBq/m² and Pu-239, -240: 4.3 kBq/m²).[8] Since reported values of Cs-137 contamination due to nuclear tests worldwide are in the range of 2.7–4.6 kBq/m² in areas located between 50 and 70 degrees latitude north,[7] we concluded that the amount of Cs-

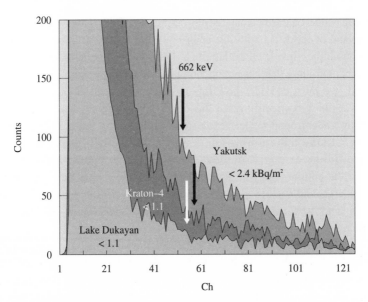

Fig. 5.9 *In-situ* γ-ray spectra around K-4 and in Yakutsk City for 30–60 min. The spectrum for Lake Dukayan was taken 100 m from the lakeside. Cs-137 contamination of the ground surface was below the detectable limits which are shown in the figure.
[From J. Takada et al., *J. Rad. Res.*, **40**, 223 (1999)]

137 surface contamination above the K-4 epicenter (underground) was normal, at least when measurements were done in March 1998.

Spectroscopy was conducted on elk flesh (15 kg), a local foodstuff of Teya village. The elk, which is a herbivorous animal, eats water grass, tree bark and lichen. Therefore, this measurement would reflect radioactive transfer among soil, plant and animal. However, the spectrum did not show a peak of Cs-137 γ-ray for 25 min. This indicates that Cs-137 contamination of the flesh was less than the detectable limit of 20 Bq/kg. This result also supports the low level of Cs-137 contamination on the ground around the K-4 hypocenter.

The present results of the radiological survey around the K-4 hypocenter confirmed that the surface of the ground was normal in 1998. In other words, the data suggested that there had been no remarkable leakage of radioactivity from the epicenter (560 m in depth) to the surface at least for non-rare gas elements as of 1998. The plutonium, fission products and radioactivity due to the explosion are likely stored in perennially frozen rocks of thickness of more than 500 m in this area.[13]

5.5 Underground Radioactivity of Kraton-4

How much and how radioactive are the materials stored underground after a nuclear explosion? Also, how are they stored and how do they affect the radiological environment in the long term? These are important questions that must be answered for radiation hygiene of the population. It is estimated from the

20-kiloton value of the nuclear fission output that Cs-137 of 88 TBq is present underground of the K-4 explosion point in 1998.[14] Sr-90 radioactivity must also exist at about the same level as that of Cs-137, although perhaps somewhat lower. Of course, plutonium that has not undergone fission also remains underground.

Next, we must consider how this radioactivity is distributed underground. There is a theory concerning the gas cavity and chimney structure which are formed by underground nuclear explosions described by the U.S. Department of Defense.[3] Using this information, a rough radioactivity distribution can be imagined. In the case of K-4, the diameter of the gas cavity is 40–60 m. The length of the chimney may be 250 m. Therefore, the radioactive material which exists underground reaches a depth of approximately 300 m below the surface of the earth in the shallowest place. At this thickness, radiation is shielded by rock and strata.

This area is a perennially frozen soil zone with an annual average temperature of minus 10°C. The thickness of the frozen soil is 500 m or more around Yakutsk. At this depth underground water does not exist. Therefore, it is difficult to conceive of leakage of radioactive material in a place deeper than 300 m to the

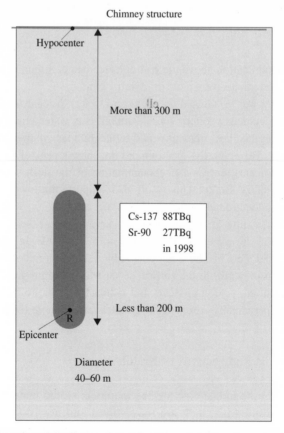

Fig. 5.10 The estimated distribution of the radioactive material from the nuclear explosion of Kraton-4.

surface of the earth via underground water. That is, the thick frozen layer confines a huge amount of radioactive material within a limited space underground.

5.6 Summary

Nuclear explosions for industrial applications were conducted in the 20th century, leaving very severe nuclear pollution underground and on the earth's surface. Long-term safety management is needed due to the long half-life of Pu-239 (24,000 y). Large amounts of fission products underground or near the surface are sources of nuclear pollution in the environment. Such explosions do not benefit society but leave behind a negative legacy for generations to come.

REFERENCES

1. United Nations Scientific Committee on the Effects of Atomic Radiation, Sources and Effects of Ionizing Radiation, *UNSCEAR 1993 Report to the General Assembly, with Scientific Annexes*, United Nations, New York (1993).
2. Soviet PNEs, A Legacy of Contamination, V. Larin, E. Tar, Bul., *Atomic Scientists*, May/June 18-20 (1999).
3. US Department of Defense, *The Effects of Nuclear Weapons* (1977).
4. V. Larin, E. Tar, Soviet, PNEs, *The Bulletin of Atomic Scientists*, May/June 18-20 (1999).
5. *Nuclear Test Explosions, SCOPE59*, John Wiley & Sons, Chichester (2000).
6. J. Takada, M. Hoshi, M. Yamamoto, T. Nagatomo, T. Imanaka, B.I. Gusev, K.N. Apsalikov, N.J. Tchaijunusova, *Health Phys.*, **73**, 524 (1997).
7. V. Yakimets, in: *Nuclear Encyclopedia*, pp.211-212, Yaroshinskaya Foundation, Moscow (in Russian) (1996).
8. G.I. Mretsky, A.S. Cyganov, S.V. Bylinkin, A.O. Popov, P.V. Ramzaev, V.V. Chugunov, *Proceedings of the Third Int. Conf. on Environmental Radioactivity in the Arctic*, pp.152-155, Tromsф, Norway (1997).
9. A.D. Gedeonov, I.N. Kuleshova, E.R. Petrov, M.L. Savopulo, B.N. Shkroev, V.G. Alexeev, V.I. Arkhipov, I.S. Burtsev, *J. Radioanal. Nucl. Chem.*, **221**, 85 (1997).
10. J. Takada, V.E. Stepanov, D.P. Yefremov, T. Shintani, A. Akiyama, M. Fukuda, M. Hoshi, *J. Rad. Res.*, **40**, 223 (1999).
11. I.A. Andryshin, V.V. Bogdan, S.A. Vashchinkin, S.A. Zelentsov, *USSR Nuclear Weapons Tests and Peaceful Nuclear Explosions 1949 through 1990*, Russian Federal Nuclear Center- VNIIEF (1996).
12. U.S. Department of Energy Nevada Operations Office of External Affairs, *United States Nuclear Tests July 1945 through September 1992*, DOE/NV-209 (Rev. 14) (1994).
13. M. Fukuda, *Arctic Siberia*, Iwanami Shoten, Tokyo (1996) (in Japanese).
14. J. Takada, K.Sh. Zumagiryov, V.E. Stepanov, T. Imanaka, T. Takatsuji, Y. Ootsuka, M. Yamamoto, I. Yoshikawa, M. Hoshi, *Radiological Investigation in the Ground Zero, Proceedings of the 3rd Workshop on Environmental Radioactivity*, KEK Proceedings 2002-7 Tsukuba, March 5-7 (2002).

6

Strict Control Zone after the Chernobyl Accident

The worst nuclear power plant accident of the 20th century occurred in Chernobyl 100 km north of Kiev in the Ukrainian Republic on April 26th, 1986. This accident caused a chain reaction of fear all over the world with the global spread of radioactive material. What are the real effects on human health and the environment? In order to understand these questions qualitatively and quantitatively studies were conducted for over 10 years after the accident. In this chapter, we focus on the strict control zone with high levels of radioactivity and review the Chernobyl accident. The investigation is ongoing.

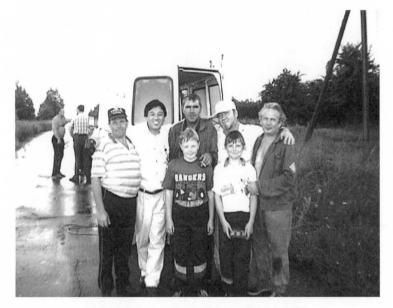

Fig. 6.1 Strict control zone, Zaborie village, in 1997.

6.1 Historical Review of the Chernobyl Nuclear Disaster[1]

The No.4 Chernobyl Nuclear Power Plant north of Kiev exploded at 1:24 a.m. on

April 26, 1986. The staff was conducting a safety test on the nuclear reactor from the previous day, and the plant was operating with the emergency cooling unit switch off. The workers tried to regain control of the crashing nuclear reactor until 1:23:40 a.m., but failed. They then attempted to insert control rods into the reactor but this also failed. The explosion occurred at 1:24. Repeated explosions continued for 10 days, and huge amounts of radioactive material were released into the atmosphere. The reactor did not have a storage container to prevent the leakage of radioactivity into the environment. The released radioactivity of 2 EBq was approximately 500 times that of the nuclear bomb dropped on Hiroshima.

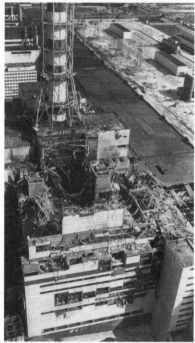
[Photo: ©Reuter/Kyodo]

Fig. 6.2 The No.4 Chernobyl nuclear reactor after the accident.

A member of the staff of the Ministry of Health telephoned the hospital of the Institute of Biophysics in Moscow at 3:14. He informed the hospital of the accident at Chernobyl and of victims with heat wounds and the possibility of radiation disease. Dr. L.A. Ilyin, Director of the Institute of Biophysics decided to send an emergency medical team to Chernobyl. The team arrived in Pripyat at 14:30. The most severely affected, 129 firemen, were sent to No.6 Hospital, Radiation Medicine Center of the Institute of Biophysics, in two airplanes on April 27.

The initial examination of the victims showed that about 30 had suffered fatal doses. Although they were still alive the radiation proved lethal despite the best efforts of the physicians. Many of the victims had hyperemia on substantial areas of the body surface, indicating a high level of exposure of skin and adjacent

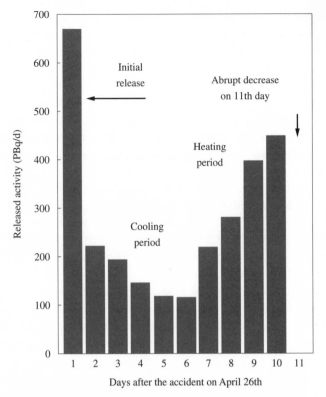

Fig. 6.3 Radioactivity released from the Chernobyl nuclear power plant accident.
[From Atomic Energy Bureau of Science Technology Agency (Japan), *Chernobyl* (1995)]

tissues. This was evidence of exposure to high doses of radiation. The firemen had worked on the roof to extinguish flames to keep them from spreading to the No.3 reactor. They wore no personal dosimeters or any radiation protection devices.

Information on the dose suffered by each victim was necessary to establish treatment. Biological dosimetry methods based on the identification of chromosomal disorder in the lymphocytes of peripheral blood and bone marrow cells were used. Whole-body dose was estimated to be 1–14 Gy. Sodium 24, which shows neutron exposure, was not detected in the radioactivity measurement in blood. Radiation disease was the primary cause of death in 17 of the 28 deceased.

A government accident investigation committee was put in place on April 26. The committee determined that the projected dose in Pripyat city 3 km from the nuclear reactor exceeded the level requiring emergency evacuation (250 mSv external dose in the USSR). This necessitated the evacuation of 45,000 citizens. The evacuation began at 2 p.m., on April 27 and was completed within three hours.

As a result of evacuation, the quantity of radioactive iodine inhaled by the inhabitants decreased. Moreover, since the inhabitants had been taking potassium iodine regularly, the effect of radioactive iodine on the thyroid was reduced. The

USSR had installed a special dosimeter around the nuclear power plant in 1976. According to the dosimeter installed in Pripyat and checked on May 3-4, the dose from this accident was 500 mSv. This indicates that the evacuation of the citizens on April 27 was effective for reducing exposure to radiation.

7,809 residents in a 10-km zone were evacuated from 10 am to 7 pm on May 3. Evacuation of 42,000 residents of the 30-km zone started the following day. 300 buses and 1100 trucks were used for this purpose. 13,000 cows and 3,000 pigs were also evacuated at the same time. These evacuations were completed on May 6. Control stations were set up at the 30-km boundary on May 3 to prevent entry of unauthorized individuals.

The maximum external dose was estimated to be 0.75 Gy for Tolsty, Stigorovka and Kopati within the 10-km zone. If evacuation had been conducted as early as the one for Pripyat city, the dose for the residents could have been reduced further. Moreover, in addition to the fact that the consumption of milk produced within the 30-km zone was not prohibited, the inhabitants had not been taking iodine for preventive purpose.

As a result, the residents of the zone received high doses in the thyroid due to the Chernobyl disaster. The average thyroid dose for children less than 18 years old in Khoyniki village and Bragin village towards Belarus was estimated to be

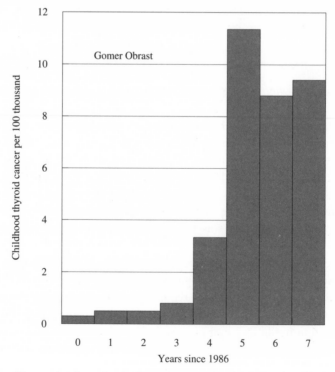

Fig. 6.4 Thyroid cancer in infants after the Chernobyl accident.
[From G.N. Souchkevitch, A.F. Tsyb, eds., *Health Consequences of the Chernobyl Accident*, WHO (1996)]

3.2 and 2.2 Gy, respectively. Among children under seven who had been evacuated early from Pripyat city, the average dose was 0.44 Gy. For adults the value was 0.15 Gy.

The occurrence of malignant tumors aside from thyroid cancer has not been confirmed so far in the population. The incidence of infant thyroid cancer increased after the accident and reached maximum in 1996. The incidence of thyroid cancer among adults is lower than among children, but it continues to rise in 2000. The incidence among women is slightly higher than among men.[4]

6.2 The 30-km Zone around Chernobyl in 1996

Environmental radiation in the 30-km zone and the strict control settlement outside of the zone in Belarus was investigated as part of the Chernobyl-Sasagawa Project in April 1996. This field investigation made possible *in-situ* measurements of cesium-137 (Cs-137) contamination density on the ground by portable γ-ray spectroscopy using an inch size NaI detector.[5] This device was calibrated using the known value of Cs-137 activity for each settlement during this project.

The shelter of the No.4 accident reactor was monitored by a team 800-member strong. No.1 and 3 reactors were still in operation (These were stopped in December 2000). γ-Ray dose rate was also measured at several sites. A dose rate of 18 μSv/h was detected about 100 m from the No.4 reactor.

There is a control disposal area for polluted trucks which had been used for clean-up after the accident. About 600 radioactive vehicles are stored in the area. The pollution remained high 10 years later. The γ dose rate was 120 μGy/h on a crane covered with soil. We can imagine how high the radiation must have been while work was being done just after the accident. According to the report by Ilyin given at the Chernobyl-Sasagawa final symposium in May 2001, the average dose in 226,900 recovery workers was 100 mSv, increasing the risk of leukemia and other cancers.[4]

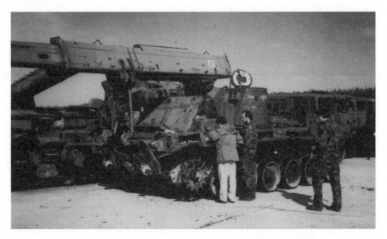

Fig. 6.5 Polluted cranes used for clean-up after the accident.

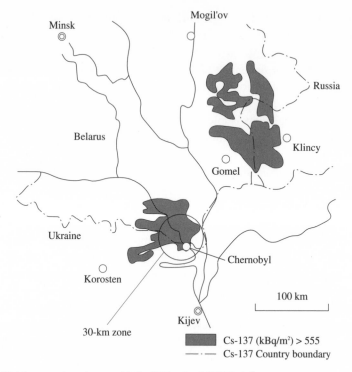

Fig. 6.6 Highly contaminated areas with Cs-137 levels of 555 kBq/m² or more.
[From *Surface Contamination Maps, Distribution of Surface Ground Contamination by Caesium-137 Released in the Chernobyl Accident and Deposited in the Byelorussian SSR,* IAEA (1989)]

The radioactive contamination was not uniform throughout the zone, as shown in Figs. 6.6 and 6.7. Areas showing levels of over 555 kBq/m² and those showing over 1,480 kBq/m² both required inhabitants to move out of the area by law. Those living in the latter were forcibly moved out while those in the former were told that it was their lawful duty to do so.

In Guden village the dose rate was 0.19 μSv/h with Cs-178 of 37–185 kBq/m². The highest dose rate was observed between Perki and Kryki in the Belarusian zone. The values are higher than the detectable limit of 19.99 μSv/h. In this area there was supposed to be no inhabitants. However, our team met a 45-year-old man who lived there with his wife. He had returned to his home land from Bryansk in 1991.

There were 56 people in Opatiti village, which is in the strict control zone. The population there before the accident was 300. A woman we met had returned in 1994. They have electric power. Living in such areas is illegal, but the government looks the other way.

The external dose in a work day for the Belarusian and Ukrainian zones was 26 μSv with an average dose rate of 3.0 μSv/h and 7.4 μSv with an average dose rate of 0.56 μSv/h, respectively, indicating that the former is more radioactively contaminated than the latter.

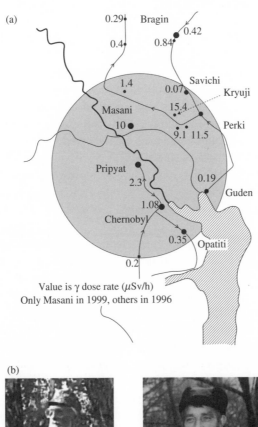

(a)

0.29 Bragin
              0.42
0.4   0.84

                  Savichi
1.4   0.07
                        Kryuji
Masani   15.4
                        Perki
10   9.1 11.5

Pripyat
      2.3   0.19
                        Guden
1.08
Chernobyl
            0.35
                  Opatiti
0.2

Value is γ dose rate (μSv/h)
Only Masani in 1999, others in 1996

(b)

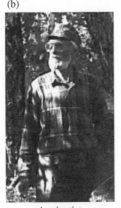

A scientist
at the Masani Radiation
Monitoring Station

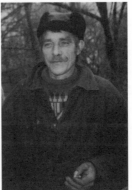

A resident of Kryuki

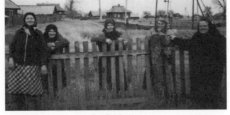

In Guden

Fig. 6.7 (a): Dose rate values in the 30-km zone around Chernobyl in 1996, and (b): related photos.

6.3 The Most Contaminated Settlement, Zaborie, Russia, in 1997

The author participated in the field mission to Bryansk Oblast in Russia with the Medical Radiation Research Center (MRRC) of Obninsk in 1997. The purpose was dosimetry studies in Zaborie, which was the most contaminated settlement in Russia. Although this village was in the strict control zone, some people live there by choice. Dosimetry studies on humans are important not only for epidemiology but also for recovery of local social activity.

Settlements showing Cs-137 doses of more than 0.56 MBq/m^2 were evacuated by the government after the Chernobyl nuclear power plant accident in 1986. However, tens of thousands of people continue to live in these settlements voluntarily.[8]

We conducted field measurements using a mobile laboratory with four spectrometers and the author's portable laboratory. This was the first time a portable system of *in-situ* spectroscopy was used for ground and whole-body counting.

. As noted above, studies on dosimetry on inhabitants are important not only for epidemiology but also for recovery of local social activity. Much previous research effort has been devoted to dose reconstruction within the framework of health effects investigations. Here we focus on dosimetry studies on individuals living in the evacuated settlements. We report estimations of whole-body external and internal accumulated doses for the period 1986-1996 and the expected doses for the years 1997-2047. The calculated doses were compared with dose estimations based on the results of ESR teeth enamel dosimetry.

6.3.1   Field Work[9]

The field mission to Zaborie [(530' 05"(N), 310' 42"(E)], the Russian territory most highly contaminated by the Chernobyl accident, conducted a dosimetry study on the residents in July 1997 (Fig. 6.1). The surface contamination was measured *in situ* using a calibrated portable NaI spectrometer (Hamamatsu C-3475) which

Table 6.1 Radiological status in and around Zaborie 1997

#	Place	Coordinates		Cs-137 (MBq/m^2)	Dose rate (μSv/h)
		N	E		
1	Makarichi Zaborie	53 04.22	31 37.15	0.33 (0.02)	0.36
2	Textile factory	53 05.04	31 42.28	4.4 (0.9)	4.40
3	Poultry farm	53 05.09	31 42.02	6.3 (1.3)	4.50
4	Hog farm	53 06.37	31 40.55	1.2 (0.1)	0.76
5	Middle of village	53 05.43	31 41.46	2.2 (0.4)	2.35
6	Barsuky	53 07.24	31 44.31	4.6 (0.3)	1.94
7	Borky	53 09.11	31 44.33	3.0 (0.6)	3.15
8	Nikolaevka	53 11.19	31 26.02	2.0 (0.4)	2.50

[Reproduced with permission from J. Takada et al., *Applied Radiation and Isotopes*, **52**, 1166 (2000) ©Elsevier Science]

has an NaI scintillator (2.5ϕ cm × 5.1 cm) and a multi channel analyzer with 128 channels (Takada 1997). The dose rate was measured by a pocket survey meter (Aloka PDR-101) in which a CsI (Tl) (20 × 25 × 15 mm) detector was installed. The local contamination of the soil was measured as being 1.5–6.3 MBq/m^2 of Cs-

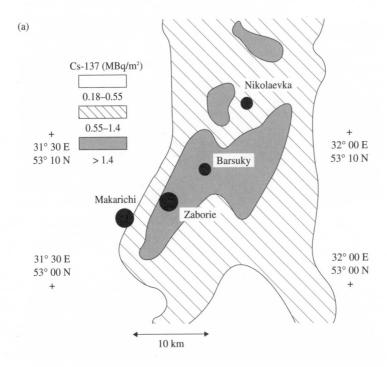

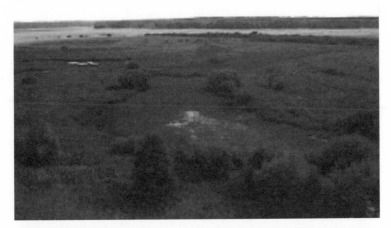

Fig. 6.8 (a) Map showing the location of Zaborie for dosimetry study with data of Cs-137 surface contamination published in map of N-36-B (1989). (b) View of Zaborie from Makarichi in 1997.
[(a): From State Committee of Geodesy and Cartography Moscow, *Map on Radiological State in the Territory of European Part of USSR of December 1989*, N-36-B (1990)]

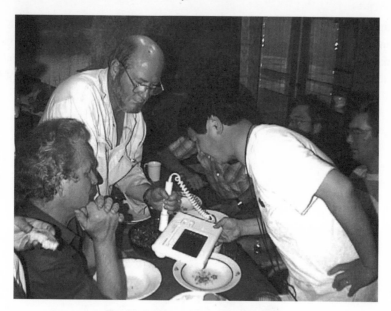

Fig. 6.9 A dinner with Cs-137 mushrooms.

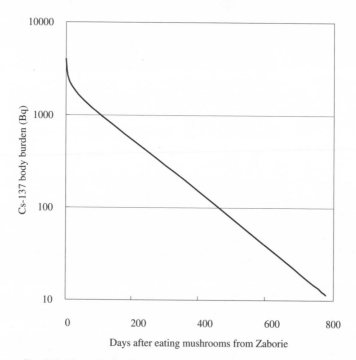

Fig. 6.10 Change in Cs-137 body burden after the dinner with mushrooms.

137 with a dose rate of 0.7–4 μSv/h.

We focused on one farmer (Case U) as a case study. Mr. U was 40 years old at the time and living in the village. We measured Cs-137 activity in the body for internal dose estimation and the environmental dose rate inside (0.7 μSv/h) and outside (2.9 μSv/h) his house for external dose estimation.

For comparison, we estimated doses on a short-term Japanese visitor to this village. This man Case T, aged 43, stayed in highly contaminated territories of the Bryansk region for nine days. He ate not only commercial food but also local fresh food, e.g., mushrooms, apples and raspberries, from the evacuated area. Cs-137 activity of the mushroom at ~ 1 kBq per piece (spectroscopic measurements) was much higher than in the other foodstuffs.

Whole-body count of Cs-137 indicated 103 kBq for Case U and 3.7 kBq for Case T. Case U was measured by a NaI spectrometer installed in the mobile laboratory of MRRC. Retention of cesium for Case T was measured by three spectrometers in Bryansk and in Hiroshima, Japan, over a period of 175 days. Half the body amount of Cs-137 in Case T decayed out within 10 days. Total biological half-life was estimated to be 104 d.

6.3.2 Estimation of Prospective Dose from 1997 to 2047

We attempted to estimate the prospective external dose $H_{extacc50}$ for Case U for 50 years beginning in 1997. The external dose rate (1.8 μSv/h) was simply assumed to be the average value inside and outside his house assuming equal time spent in each. We assumed the main component of accidental radioactivity to be Cs-137 since the activity of Cs-134 is negligibly small for long-term estimation after 1997. Moreover, it was assumed that the annual dose H_{extan} subtracted from the natural background value (0.11 μSv/h) decreased with the physical half-life of Cs-137, with depth migration into the ground and a snow shielding factor of 0.9. The annual external dose H_{extani}(external-annual-i) in i-th year from 1997 can be expressed by

$$H_{extani} = H_{extano}(0.5)^{i/T_p} (0.5)^{i/T_d} \qquad (6.1)$$

where H_{extano} = 13.32 mSv/y in 1997, T_p = 30.0 y is half-life of Cs-137 and T_d = 50.0 y is half-time of depth migration of Cs-137 (MU 2.6.1.-96.).[11]

Figure 6.11 shows the long-term dynamics of Cs-137 annual external dose calculated using equation (6.1). Then we obtain $H_{extacc50}$ (external accumulate in 50 years) = 269 mSv/50y for Case U over 50 years by

$$H_{extacc50} = 0.87 \sum_{i=0}^{49} H_{extani} \qquad (6.2)$$

where the time-averaged shielding factor of the house for "soft" γ-rays is calculated to be 0.87 (MU 2.6.1.-96.).

Next we assume the following simple model for the internal dose for 50 years.

People in the village eat local contaminated foodstuffs. Cs-137 activity in Case U's body is I_0' in summer of the first year (1997) and $(1-a) I_0'$ in winter. Then

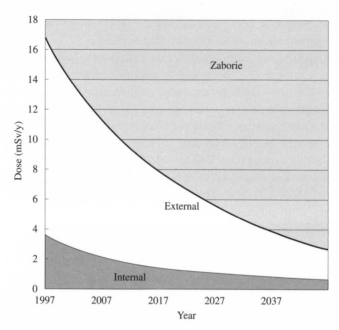

Fig. 6.11 Long-term dynamics of the annual dose from Cs-137 in Zaborie.

average Cs-137 activity of the body in the first year becomes $I_0 = I_0' (1 - 0.5a)$. The value of a is assumed to be 0.06 for Zaborie. The difference between the summer and winter periods came from the difference in the kinds of food ingested by cattle and poultry during the winter and summer periods. As a result the concentration of cesium in the human body during winter is different by a factor of $(1-a)$ compared with that in summer. The value of a was estimated based on large-scale whole-body counting in winter and summer for the population in the contaminated territories, i.e., residents who were living continuously in the contaminated Bryansk region. Average Cs-137 activity I_i of the body in the i-th year is

$$I_i = I_0 \times 0.5^{i/T_f} \tag{6.3}$$

where $I_0 = 99.9$ kBq for Case U, and T_f is the effective half-life of Cs-137 intake due to local foodstuffs for local inhabitants after 1994. In the calculation, we assumed the two values of 7.1 y and 30 y for T_f.[11,12] These values were reported for Belarus and Russian territories, respectively. Zaborie is located in the western part of Russia, near the boundary between Belarus and Russia.

The annual dose can be calculated by

$$H_{intani} = 0.0352\ I_i\ (mSv/y) \tag{6.4}$$

where I_i is in kBq. In this formula, we assume an annual limit of intake of Cs-137

(4MBq) of ICRP30 and a biological half-life ($T_{b1/2}$) of 100 d. If the value of $T_{b1/2}$, which is reported to be between 50 and 150 days, is assumed to be 110 days, the coefficient of eq. (6.4) increases about 10%. The long-term dynamics of Cs-137 annual internal dose calculated using eq. (6.4) is shown in Fig. 6.11.

Then the internal dose H_{int50} for 50 years is estimated to be between 38 and 106 mSv/50y by

$$H_{int50} = \sum_{i=0}^{49} H_{intanni} \tag{6.5}$$

For the short-term visitor from Japan to this area, the external and internal doses were estimated to be 0.13 mSv/9d and 0.024 mSv/50y, making the total dose 0.15 mSv/50y due to the short stay in this highly contaminated territory.

6.3.3 Doses during 1986-1996

Accumulated external doses for the period 1986-1996 may be calculated according to the model presented in MU 2.6.1.-96.[11] The estimate is 130 mSv for Zaborie where Cs-137 contamination was assumed to be 3.7 MBq/m^2.

Moreover, wide-scale ESR-teeth enamel measurements in contaminated Bryansk settlements were used to estimate mean values of accumulated dose for the inhabitants of Zaborie. About 2,500 measurements were carried out on tooth enamel samples collected in radioactively contaminated territories of the Bryansk region.[13] To avoid the effect of solar light only back teeth were used. The methods of sample preparation, dose measurements as well as values of correction factors were reported earlier.[14,15] Correction factor on the energy dependence of enamel sensitivity, age dependence due to natural background radiation as well as the value of initial intrinsic signal were taken into account for more correct dose estimation. Since no teeth samples were available for Zaborie village, the results of measurements from more than 20 other contaminated Bryansk settlements were used for external dose reconstruction of Zaborie. These studies showed that the average ESR-teeth enamel dose has a tendency to grow with the levels of Cs-137 contamination of settlements:

$$D = b^* q_{Cs} \tag{6.6}$$

where b = (0.065 +/-0.013) mGy per kBq/m^2; q_{Cs} = mean contamination density of the soil by Cs-137, kBq/m^2; D = accumulated dose over 10 years after the accident. The b value in eq. (6.6) was estimated based on large-scale ESR teeth enamel dosimetry investigations in the Bryansk region and represents the result of regression analysis of ESR teeth enamel dose (D) versus Cs-137 (q_{Cs}) contamination of the settlements from which the samples of teeth were collected. For Zaborie village, in a place with contamination of 3.7 MBq/m^2, the corresponding calculation gives the value 240 mGy ± 50 mGy. Taking into account the efficiency of the countermeasures taken in Zaborie against external irradiation (25%), the final value equals 180 ± 37 mGy. It should be noted that some additional input to teeth dose due to irradiation by β particles of Cs-137 from soft tissue of the mouth is possible. This factor is currently under investigation.

The mean value of accumulated Cs-137, -134 internal dose for adults in Zaborie in the 10 years after the Chernobyl accident was estimated to be 16 mSv taking into account the official countermeasures (e.g., replacing contaminated milk with uncontaminated milk) just after the accident established by the government.[11]

Table 6.2   Doses in Zaborie

Period	Effective dose (mSv)	
	1986-1996	1997-2047
Internal	16	72
External	130[*1] or 180[*2]	269

[*1] Value calculated by the model presented in
     MU 2.6.1-96.[11]
[*2] Value estimated using data based on wide-
     scale ESR-teeth enamel measurements in
     contaminated Bryansk settlements
[Reproduced with permission from J. Takada
et al., *Applied Radiation and Isotopes*, **52**,
1168 (2000) ©Elsevier Science]

6.4 Intervention of the Former USSR for Radiation Protection of the Inhabitants[7]

The basic plan for the radiological protection of the public in an emergency situation involving a large-scale nuclear disaster is formulated in peacetime. However, various problems seem to have occurred at the actual time of intervention. Criteria for urgent decision making in the event of an accidental release of radioactivity into the environment was developed in the former USSR in the 1960s. After that, the plan had been revised in three times, and approved by the Ministry of Health in August 1983. Immediately after the Chernobyl accident, some measure of protection was taken based on this document. These decisions included evacuation of the town of Pripyat as well as decisions regarding prophylaxis using iodine and the evacuation of other settlements within a 30-km zone. The decisions were made based on the estimation of radiation levels which showed the possibility of exceeding criteria levels by external gamma radiation and inhalation of radioiodine.

The USSR Academy of Science proposed a new concept regarding average annual effective dose. When the average annual effective dose due to the radioactive pollution by fallout exceeds 1 mSv, general protection measures must be executed to prevent the level from exceeding 5 mSv.

After termination of the period of radioiodine hazard, for implementation of measures to protect the population for external and internal radiation by Cs-137,

Table 6.3 Criteria for making decisions on measures to protect the population in the event of a reactor accident in the former USSR (approved August 4, 1983)

Nature of exposure	Level of exposure	
	A	B
External γ radiation (Gy)	0.25	0.75
Thyroid exposure due to intake of radioactive iodine (Gy)	0.25-0.30	2.5
Integrated concentration of I-131 in air (kBq s/l)		
Children	1,480	14,800
Adults	2,590	25,900
Total intake of I-131 with food (kBq)	55.5	555
Maximum contamination by I-131 of fresh milk (kBq/l), or of daily food intake (kBq/d)	3.7	37
Initial I-131 fallout density in pasture (kBq/m^2)	25.9	259

If exposure or contamination does not exceed level A, there is no need to take emergency measures that involve the temporary disruption of the normal life routine of the public.

If exposure or contamination exceeds level A but does not reach level B, it is recommended that decisions be taken on the basis of the actual situation and local conditions.

If exposure or contamination reaches or exceeds level B, it is recommended that emergency measures be taken to ensure protection of the public from radiation: the public should immediately seek shelter indoors; time spent outdoors should be restricted: on the basis of the actual situation, rapid evacuation should be organized; prophylactic iodine should be distributed; the use of contaminated products in food banned or limited; dairy cattle should be moved to uncontaminated pasture or fodder.

[Reproduced with permission from Yu.O. Konstantinov, *Decision Making on Population Protection in a Large-scale Radioactive Contamination Following a Nuclear Reactor Accident, Proceedings of the Russian-Hungarian Seminar on Radiation Protection, Budapest 1991* (1992)]

pollution density was accepted as the criterion for zoning the territories according to levels of predicted radiation exposure of the population.

Protective and social measures were implemented in the territories with surface contamination $W > 37$ kBq/m^2 or an excess of the effective annual dose for 1991, $D > 1$ mSv. A territory where $W = 185–555$ kBq/m^2 is designated as a zone whose inhabitants have the right to relocate. A territory with $W > 555$ kBq/m^2 is a zone of relocation, including compulsory relocation if $W > 1,480$ kBq/m^2 or $D > 5$ mS.

As a result of such protection measures, external dose of the public should not exceed 250–750 mSv. The thyroid dose of most residents did not exceed the regulation value. However, since the protection measures were not applied successfully to those who resided in the areas part-time, the thyroid dose exceeded the standard level. The maximum for infants reached several Sieverts.

For social, psychological and political reasons, great efforts to minimize the discrepancy between scientifically prepared standards and actual application are demanded. To apply theory to society, much preparation is necessary. In the case of Chernobyl, there was an overwhelming lack of equipment for monitoring and use of iodine for preventive purposes.

6.5 Summary

The characteristics of the radiation exposure of the population in the Chernobyl nuclear power plant accident are summarized as follows.

1) Huge quantities of radioactivity of about 2 EBq were released into the environment.

2) 95,000 residents in the 30-km zone were evacuated between the 2nd and 7th day after the accident. This reduced the dose effectively. However, the maximum dose equivalent and thyroid dose were estimated to be 750 mSv and several Sv, respectively.

3) Intervention for thyroid-protection was implemented only for the population of Prypiat and not carried out for other populations. The consumption of milk which was produced in the 30-km zone was not prohibited. Iodine potassium was not prepared for populations other than that of Prypiat. This led to a maximum dose of several Sv for thyroid.

4) A wide area of land was polluted with radioactive materials of long half-life. Especially in areas where rain fell while the radioactive cloud was passing, pollution by Cs-137 was remarkable. The total area which was polluted to a level of 555 kBq/m^2 or more in the three countries of Russia, Belarus and Ukraine was 10,300 km^2. This is 4.7 times the area of Tokyo.

5) Areas polluted by Cs-137(W) at levels of 555 kBq/m^2 or more were designated relocation zones, including compulsory relocation if they indicated W >1,480 kBq/m^2 or an annual dose > 5 mSv. Such areas are designated as the strict control zone. The annual dose 10 years after the accident was at a level of several mSv for people in the strict control zone.

6) Because there are adults who live in the strict control zone by choice, the author believes that long-term investigation and support for revival of the zone are necessary.

REFERENCES

1. L.A. Ilyn, *Chernobyl: Myth and Reality*, Alara Limited, Moscow (1994).
2. Atomic Energy Bureau of the Science Technology Agency (Japan), *Chernobyl* (1995) (in Japanese).
3. G.N. Souchkevitch, A.F. Tsyb, eds., *Health Consequences of the Chernobyl Accident*, World Health Organization, Geneva (1996).
4. L.A. Ilyn, *Radiation Accidents: Medical Effects and Radiation Protection Experience, Chernobyl: Message for the 21st Century. Proc. of the Sixth Chernobyl Sasakawa Medical Cooperation Symposium, Moscow, 2001*, 7-17, Elsevier (2002).
5. J. Takada, Y. Ogino, S. Tani, S. Endo, Y. Nitta, M. Hoshi, H. Stow, T. Takatsuji, I. Yoshikawa, V.B. Masyakin, V.F. Sharifov, I.V. Pilenko, I.I. Veselkina, *Jpn. J. Med Phys. Suppl.*, **51**, 31 (1997) (in Japanese).
6. The International Chernobyl Project (1991), *Surface Contamination Maps, Distribution of Surface Ground Contamination by Caesium-137 Released in the Chernobyl Accident and Deposited in the Byelorussian SSR*, the Russian SFSR and

the Ukrainian SSR (December 1989), IAEA.

7. Yu.O. Konstantinov, *Decision Making on Population Protection in a Large-scale Radioactive Contamination Following a Nuclear Reactor Accident, Proceedings of the Russian-Hungarian Seminar on Radiation Protection, Budapest 1991* (1992).

8. Yu.A. Izrael, E.V. Kvasnikova, I.M. Nazarov, Sh.D. Fridman, *Meteorology and Hydrology*, No.5, 5-9 (1994) (in Russian).

9. J. Takada, M. Hoshi, S. Endo, V.F. Stepanenko, A.E. Kondrashov, D. Petin, V. Skvortsov, A. Ivannikov, D. Tikounov, Y. Gavrilin, V.P. Snykov, *Applied Radiation and Isotopes*, **52**, 1165 (2000).

10. State Committee of Geodesy and Cartography Moscow, *Map on Radiological State in the Territory of European Part of USSR of December 1989*, N-36-B (Gomel), 1990 (in Russian).

11. MU 2.6.1.-96. *"Reconstruction of Mean Accumulated dose in 1986-1995 Effective Dose of Irradiation of the Inhabitants of Rusian's Settlements Which Were Contaminated following the Accident in Chernobyl NPP in 1986."* Methodical Directions, Official Issue, Goskomsanepidnadzor, Russia, Moscow (1996) (in Russian).

12. Ministry of Health of Belarus Republic., *Methodical Directions*, *"The Prognosis of Annual Effective Dose of Irradiation of Inhabitants of the Belarus Republic's Settlements,"* Minsk (1995) (in Russian).

13. A.I. Ivannikov, V.G. Skvortsov, V.F. Stepanenko, D.D. Tikunov, I.M. Fedosov, A.A. Romanjukha, A. Wieser, *Radiat. Prot. Dosim.*, **71** (3), 175 (1997).

14. V.G. Skvortsov, A.I. Ivannikov, U. Eichhoff, *J. Molec. Struct.*, **347**, 321 (1995).

15. V. Stepanenko, V. Skvortsov, A. Tsyb, A. Ivannikov, A. Kondrashov, D. Tikunov, E. Iaskova, V. Shakhtarin, D. Petin, E. Parshkov, I. Chernichenko, V. Snykov, M. Orlov, Yu. Gavrilin, V. Khrousch, S. Shinkarev, *Radiat. Prot. Dosim.*, **77**, No. 1/2, 101 (1998).

7

Radiation Exposure of the Population in the Tokaimura Criticality Accident

In 1999, a criticality accident occurred in Tokaimura, Japan, a center for research and development of nuclear technology for peaceful purposes. This level-4 accident did not cause any long-term physical hazards, but it had a strong psychological impact on society. The author, who had been working in the strict control zone of Belarus at the time of this accident, went to investigate Tokaimura immediately after returning to Japan. In this chapter, we mainly verify the dose of exposure to the public by this accident.

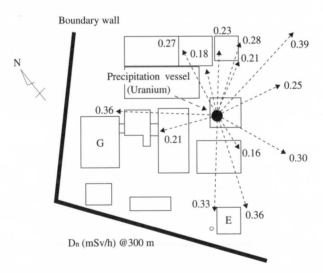

Fig. 7.1 Vector expression of the neutron dose rate. The value, which was measured by a rem counter between 19:09 and 19:22, September 30, 1999, was normal at a distance of 300 m.

7.1 A Brief Review of the Tokaimura Criticality Accident

Japan's greatest nuclear power disaster occurred on September 30, 1999, at Tokaimura located 135 km northeast of Tokyo.[1] The accident occurred while three workers were manufacturing 18.8% enriched uranyl nitrate solution as nuclear fuel for the experimental fast breeder reactor, Joyo, of the Japan Nuclear Cycle Development Institute (JNC) in a conversion facility of the uranium fuel processing factory of JCO Co., Ltd., from the previous day.[2]

A nuclear fission chain reaction occurs in nuclear fuel when radioactive material reaches critical mass. The handling and management of nuclear fuel must therefore be strictly controlled based on scientific and technical principles at the processing factory. However, at the JCO factory of the Tokaimura facility, productivity took precedence over safety. The criticality accident occurred when a worker using a bucket poured uranyl solution into a precipitation vessel, dissolving 2.4 kilograms of uranium powder at 10:35 a.m. on September 30.[2] After that, the resulting criticality condition continued for 20 hours, radiating γ-rays and neutrons into the perimeter.

Two workers who saw the blue flash evacuated to a decontamination room located in an adjacent building connected by a corridor with a third man and lost consciousness. One of them contacted someone outside, an ambulance was requested from the Tokaimura Fire Department at 10:43 and the three workers were rescued. Three ambulance worker suffered external doses of between 5 and 9 mSv at this time.[3] This was determined by whole-body counting for sodium-24 (Na-24).

The three victims were transported to the National Institute of Radiological Sciences in Chiba via National Mito Hospital by helicopter. They were housed in emergency medical treatment facilities at 15:25. Physicists detected Na-24 clearly in the γ-ray spectrum for vomitus, confirming neutron exposure.

Because the workers were not wearing individual dosimeters, analysis was conducted using physical and biological methods.

The doses for the three men were estimated from the acute radiation symptoms and were 4 Grey equivalent (GyEq) or less, 6 GyEq or more and 8 Gy Eq or more, respectively. Finally, the doses were estimated to be 16–20, 6–10 and 1–4.5 GyEq, respectively, as a result of decreases in corpuscles and lymphocytes, chromosome analysis, measurement of the radioactivity in the body induced by neutrons, and other tests.[3]

Because there were no specialists for medical treatment at the National Institute of Radiological Sciences, two of the victims with high doses were moved to two hospitals of the University of Tokyo on October 2 and 4. Despite treatment including end blood stem cell transfusion, umbilical cord blood transfusion and skin grafts, the workers died of massive organ failure on the 83rd and 211th day after the accident.

The criticality accident occurred at a height of about 1 m in a one-story building. It was not an explosion, but the uranium continued undergoing nuclear fission for over 19 hours. According to evaluations by Dr. T. Mitsugashira of Tohoku University and by the Japan Atomic Energy Research Institute (JAERI), the total amount of fission of uranium-235 (U-235) was about 1 mg.[4] This is approximately one millionth of the 800 g of the Hiroshima N-bomb.

Fission products such as rare gas and iodine leaked outdoors through the exhaust port of the conversion building. However, a considerable quantity remained in the precipitate vessel. The leakage of iodine-134 (I-134) and total radioactive iodine was estimated to be about 5 GBq and 13 GBq, respectively, by JNC.[5] The total activity of I-131 released to the environment in this criticality accident was 1/900,000,000 of that of the Chernobyl accident (630 PBq). The thyroid dose was estimated to be 0.02 mSv, a very low level. The main characteristic of the Tokaimura criticality accident was external exposure by residents of the surrounding area to neutrons and γ-rays which had leaked out.

7.2 Evacuation of Residents

The Science and Technology Agency, which is responsible for the safe regulation of nuclear power, received the first report at 11:19. It was at 12 o'clock that the professional staff of the government service at Tokaimura began to grasp the state of affairs at the JCO Tokai facility. It was decided to establish a government task force at 15:00. At 17:00 a local headquarters was installed at the JAERI at Tokaimura. At 18:00 an emergency technological advisory committee meeting began and this committee sent members from Sumida and Kanagawa to Tokaimura to evaluate the situation. Their major concern was to make technological decisions to end the crisis.

Meanwhile, the Tokaimura local government, which had received a telephone call about the occurrence of the criticality accident from the JCO Tokai office at 11:33, established a headquarters at 12:15 to undertake immediate measures for radiation protection of the residents of the area. γ-Rays showed a maximum level of 0.8 mSv/h at the boundary near the accident site. At 12:30, the Tokaimura government began radio announcements informing residents of the surrounding area about the disaster and the need to seek shelter. The Tokaimura accident measure headquarters started emergency evacuation of residents living within a 350-m zone between 15:00 and 15:45.

Neutron dose was measured at boundaries of the JCO campus by rem counter from 19:09. γ-Ray and neutron dose rates were between 0.002 and 0.5 mSv/h and between 0.015 and 4.5 mSv/h, respectively. The ratio of the two kinds of radiation was about 9.

Figure 7.2 shows the values of γ-ray monitoring in the JCO factory. The output changed dramatically for 25 minutes immediately after the criticality occurred (burst period), then gradually decreased (Plateau 1 period). It remained almost constant from 20:45 to 3:30 October 1 (Plateau 1 period), then decreased to one-third after the cooling water around the precipitation vessel was drained. Finally, criticality was terminated at 6:15 October 1.

For activities such as traffic regulation around the accident site, policemen were dispatched even as the criticality continued. It lasted a maximum of 14 hours. Each officer wore an individual dosimeter. Based on the (γ-ray) dose value, we estimated neutron dose (9.2 times γ-ray) and evaluated the total dose for each officer. As a result, seven officers showed levels of 1 mSv or more, with a maximum value of 4.9 mSv. Other policemen indicated less than 1 mS.

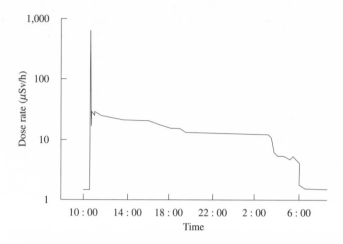

Fig. 7.2 Record of radiation monitoring during the accident. γ-Ray dose rates.
[From Nuclear Power Safety Committee, *White Paper on Nuclear Power* (2000)]

7.3 Directional Distribution of Radiation in the Residential Area

Until the protection wall of thick concrete was installed around the conversion
ridge where the uranium was located after the accident, radiation leaked out of the
site. Surveys of β- and γ-rays were carried out on the walls of the boundary and
buildings in the JCO factory at Tokaimura more than 22 days after the accident by
the author. The dose rate of leaked radiation was 0.035 μSv/h at the boundary wall
of the JCO campus on October 23. β Counts were conducted on the surface (72
cm^2) of the concrete wall. Remarkable distribution of β-rays was observed on the
wall depending on the complex internal and external structures of the building
surrounding the critical uranium (Fig. 7.3).

We observed radiation levels of more than 20 μSv/h at the wall of the
conversion ridge. The most remarkable finding was the maximal level at the outer
wall of the building adjacent to the one in which the accident occurred, which was
connected by an indoor corridor. The two sites indicating the maximum β-ray
count and the uranium source were on a single line. There was no concrete
structure between the two sites showing the maximum levels, i.e., the uranium
source and adjacent building, but there was a thin steel plate door. Neutrons had
penetrated the steel plate and leaked out strongly in the direction of the adjacent
building.

A directional distribution was mathematically derived by analyzing data of
radiation on the wall. As a result, it was found that the directional distribution of
the radiation leaked after the accident agreed with the distribution of the neutron
dose rate which was measured during criticality. This confirms that β-ray counting
can indirectly measure γ-rays from the fission products after an accident. The
fission products with the most intensive γ-ray level of 1596 keV γ-rays of
lanthanum-140 (La-140) remained mainly in the precipitation vessel. The

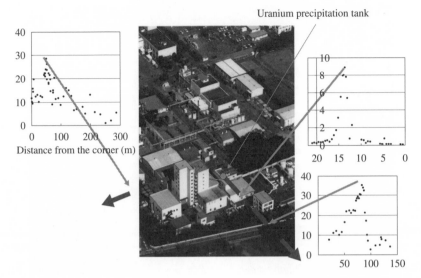

Fig. 7.3 Leakage of radiation from the uranium source after the accident October 23-26, 1999. The spatial distribution of the β-ray counts on a boundary wall and outer wall of the conversion building.
[Photo: ©Kyodo News]

directional distribution may depend on the structure and the material of the building surrounding a uranium source. The radiation leakage is greater in the direction of the thinner concrete wall. This condition may be the same during criticality. Neutrons leaked out in addition to γ-rays during the accident. The ratio between the two types of radiation was almost constant everywhere around the JCO factory. The directional distribution of radiation, which was measured after the accident, can be used as the distribution of the leakage radiation near the JCO factory during the criticality accident.

Figure 7.4 indicates the directional distribution of radiation over a photograph of the residential areas around the JCO site. The dotted line around the conversion building (○) where the uranium was located shows the radiation distribution. The radiation is strong in the direction north of this dotted line and becomes weak in the direction south of the line. However, the distribution to the east is unclear. There was no concrete wall in that direction. In the northeastern direction, the leakage radiation was weak because the site boundary was comparatively distant, and the distribution could not be measured.

There were two directions with strong radiation: one in the direction of neighboring offices to the northwest and the other in the direction of the vacant land to the southwest. The weakest radiation was in the direction of the residential neighborhood to the southwest, in the shadow of Building E of JCO. The dose is one-fifth that in the maximum direction.

For the dose reconstruction for residents in the surrounding area, the directional distribution of the radiation leaked is one of the most important pieces of information. However, the accident investigation committee only obtained dose

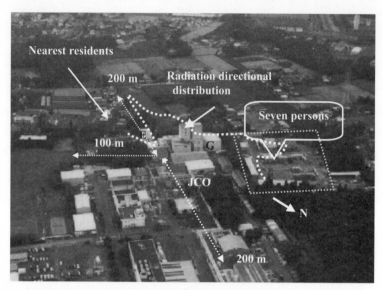

Fig. 7.4 Overview of the residential areas around the JCO accident site with a
schematic illustration of the radiation directional distribution. The radiation for
the nearest residents in the southwesterly direction was strongly shielded by
Building E and others. A mathematical expression of the radiation distribution
has been reported.
[From J. Takada, *J. Radiat. Res.*, **42**: Suppl., S77 (2001)]

evaluation of distance. Since no direct data regarding the directional distribution
during criticality was available, the directional distribution obtained indirectly
played an important role in the dose reconstruction for the residents.

7.4 External Dose to Residents within a 350-m Zone[8]

7.4.1   Facts on Dose for the Residents

The existence of anisotropic radiation from the JCO accident and the directional
distribution function in some directions has been confirmed in a previous study.[7]
Dose-rate data of neutrons which were measured at 13 sites around the boundary
of the JCO campus at 7 pm on September 30 using a rem counter clearly showed
an anisotropic feature depending on the external and internal building structures
around the uranium source. Moreover, the directional distribution function of β-
ray counts on the boundary concrete wall 880 m long after the accident was
consistent with neutron dose rate data in several directions. The nearest residential
area was in the southwesterly direction, and a remarkably steep distribution was
discovered there. The lowest relative value of the directional distribution was 0.2
in this direction. This was completely different from the isotropic radiation
released in the Hiroshima and Nagasaki atomic bomb explosions in which the
hypocenter was about 500 m high in the sky.

The directional distribution of radiation must be taken into account for the dose reconstruction of residents in the 350-m evacuated zone. However, in the official report (Head Office of Countermeasures, January 31, 2000) only the distance dependence of the dose was used as the individual dose, providing misguided information for dose reconstruction of the population.[3] Although the best solution is to use direct measurements of the dose rate at each site where a resident was located, the number of measurement sites is very limited. The first public dose in the correct direction was evaluated by using the directional distribution function and the first version of the distance dependence of dose (Head Office of Countermeasure Nov. 5, 1999).[2,9] On the other hand, individual doses were evaluated by an excellent technique for seven persons who were in a neighboring company to the west of the accident site. The Japan Nuclear Cycle Development Institute evaluated individual doses based on measurements for whole-body counts (WBC) on Na-24 for them.[10,11] This was a unique evaluation of individual doses for the public using personal data.

7.4.2 Method of Dose Reconstruction for the Residents

The external dose for person i, who was exposed to radiation between the beginning of the accident (t_0) and the time of evacuation (t_E), is expressed as

$$D_i = \int_{t_0}^{t_E} D_{ri} (r_{s.}, \theta_{s.}, t) \, dt \tag{7.1}$$

where $Dr_i (r_{s.}, \theta_{s.}, t)$ is the effective dose equivalent rate at site s and time t, and $s = \delta_i (t)$ is the site data for person i.

We applied the following approximation for the dose rate at site s:

$$Dr_i (r_s, \theta_s, t) = TF_s \, \Phi \, (\theta_s) \, D \, (r_s, t) \tag{7.2}$$

where $D (r_{s.}, t)$ is the effective dose equivalent rate (neutrons plus γ-rays) as a function of distance and time,[12] $\Phi (\theta_s)$ is the directional distribution function of radiation[7] and TF_s is the transmission factor of the house at site s.

The value of $D (r_{s.}, t)$ is the second version, which was reported on December 11, 1999, by the Head Office of Countermeasures after a reevaluation of the ratio between the burst and the plateau of criticality.[12] The value is based on the original data of 1-cm dose equivalent rate.

We assume the directional distribution function ($\phi (\theta_s)$) for radiation which was previously reported by us.[7] This was derived from a β-ray survey of the concrete walls of the JCO boundary on October 23-25. This function is consistent with the neutron dose-rate measurements at several sites. The dose-rate ratio of neutrons/γ-rays was constant at several sites. For example, the ratio for dose in Sv units was found to be 9.2 ± 1.6 at 13 sites near the boundary of the JCO factory at 7 pm on September 30.[1]

The value of $\Phi (\theta_s)$, which was applied for the dose reconstruction of residents within 350 m, was analyzed using data obtained between 80 and 200 m from the source. The function $\Phi(\theta_s)$ is more effective for residents closer to the boundary of the JCO campus. It should be noted that the residents closer to the source experienced larger doses. On the contrary, $\Phi(\theta_s)$ is ineffective for use in dose reconstruction for sites far from the boundary due to the multiple scattering of radiation.

This function has been applied to both neutrons and γ-rays based on evidence in which the dose ratio between the two kinds of radiation is almost constant (variation of less than 20%) in all directions at distances of between 80 and 500 m.[7] Fig. 7.4 shows a schematic illustration of the directional distribution of radiation in an overview of the residential areas around the JCO site. The value of $\Phi(\theta_s)$ is between 0.2 and 1.0 in the residential areas west of the source.[7] In particular, residents in the southwesterly direction, which was shielded by JCO buildings, showed low values of $\Phi(\theta_s)$. For example, the closest resident ($r = 102$ m) in this direction had a $\Phi(\theta_s)$ of 0.18.

The evaluation of TF_s for each house is the most complicated problem for dose reconstruction, since each house does not stand in free space, as shown in Fig. 7.4. The entire residential area should be treated as a three-dimensional system, especially for houses near the JCO campus. The houses far from the source may be treated as a single or a small cluster of houses according to the dominant component of irradiation from the skyshine. It is noted that the closest resident was only 102 m far from the source.

In this study, we calculated the dose under two imaginary cases for shielding in residential areas. One was an outdoor dose with $TF_s = 1.0$, which corresponds to the maximum dose at each site. However, we know that this is a rare case, because such a site on vacant land or a site along a street around the JCO campus has no shielding between the site and the boundary of the JCO campus, as shown in Fig. 7.1. Policemen who stood on the street during the accident illustrate this case. Sites in front of the nearest house in each direction also illustrate this case. On the other hand, TF_s for outdoors is not always 1.0, but less than 1.0, since some shielding also exists outdoors. For example, if a person was standing in the yard of his house, the houses between him and the source acted as a radiation shield, especially in the 350-m zone near the radiation source.

Another imaginary case would be to calculate the indoor dose with a constant value for the shielding between the site and the boundary of the JCO campus. TF_s would be 0.4 in the present simple evaluation. This value is based on a dosimetry study of the Hiroshima and Nagasaki atomic bombs. The values of TF were reported to be 0.36–0.41 and 0.42–0.43 (neutrons) and 0.54–0.52 and 0.56–0.52 (prompt γ-rays) for a single-story structure.[13] In actuality, each house has a different TF value due to the difference in structure and materials as well as the various objects inside and the various environments around each house. In any case, as noted above, the entire residential area near the JCO site, which should be treated as a three-dimensional system, poses a complicated problem. Consequently we treated TF_s as an effective transmittance for all of the houses. The TF_s value of 0.4 is an approximation.

Seven persons at a neighboring company west of the JCO campus were located at distances of 84–202 m between 10:35 and 16:00 on the day of the accident (Fig. 7.4.). They moved among several sites during this period. The site data, $s = \delta_i(t)$, for each person (i) are expressed numerically based on data from interviews with them.[11]

7.4.3   Confirmation of Dosimetry

Only sites a and f were located indoors in a small prefabricated single-story house. The other sites (b, c, d, e) were located outdoors, as shown in Fig. 7.5. Two of seven persons remained mainly indoors (site a or f) until evacuation. Three other persons remained at their site a during lunch time. All seven remained at site f for two hours just before the evacuation. The values of $\Phi(\theta_s)$ range from 0.48 to 0.81 for these sites.

TF_s for outdoor locations of this company may have been less than 1.0 since some large metallic materials were located at each working site. Indoor TF_s at sites a and f may be greater than 0.4 in this prefabricated house with thin walls. An estimation for the wall (model of 0.4 mm-thick iron plate with 12 mm-thick wood plate) gave transmittance values of 0.82 and 0.90 for neutrons and γ-rays, respectively.[3] However, objects inside as well as other human bodies no doubt reduced the transmittance effectively for each person in a small room. This particular study was not clear in the structural details.

These individual site data as a function of time were summarized as r_s, θ_s and $s = \delta_i(t)$ (a, b, c, d, e and f) for each person (i). Table 7.1 lists the site data for the seven individuals. The dose reconstruction for these seven persons were 16, 11 and 13 mSv as maximal, minimal and average values of individual effective doses (D_i), respectively.

Fifty to ninety percent of the dose for them came from indoors (sites a and f). This leads to a maximum positive error of 6 to 13 mSv (50 to 100%) for an individual dose from the error of TF_s (the maximum value corresponding to $TF_s = 0.8$). An outdoors site with some shielding also leads to a negative error of –3 mSv (–30%) at most.

The data for $s = \delta_i(t)$ were confirmed by several interviews with each person. However, each person moved within an area of several meters around the site, affecting $\phi(\theta_s)$ and $D(r_s, t)$. This would cause an ± 11% error, at maximum.

$\Phi(\theta_s)$ with ± 20% error in this area gives an error of ± 20% for the dose. The error of $D(r_s, t)$, which was reported to be ± 40%, causes an error of ± 40% for the dose. Thus total error of dose for the seven persons becomes –55% to + 110%.

These results show good coincidence with evaluations from the data on WBC of Na-24 by JNC shown in Table 7.2. The individual doses from WBC were 16, 7 and 11 mSv maximum, minimum and average values, respectively, with errors of between –23% and 58%.[3,11] The average value of the ratio between the present and JNC individual doses was 0.92 ± 0.31. This coincidence supports not only the validity of our method concerning individual dose reconstruction based on the

Table 7.1 $S = \delta i$ (t) : Site data for the seven persons

Person number	Time on Sep. 30 1999				
	10:35	12:00	13:00	14:00	16:00
W1	a	a	a	a	f
W2	a	a	a	a	f
W3	c	c	e	c	f
W4	c	c	e	c	f
W5	b	b	a	b	f
W6	d	d	a	d	f
W7	d	d	a	d	f

Site Number   a-f
W1:   out 12:10-12:30, 13:40-14:00
W2:   out 12:10-12:30
[From J. Takada, *J. Radiat. Res.*, **42**; Supple., S79 (2001)]

Table 7.2   Individual dose for seven persons

Individual dose (mSv)			
	Present	JNC	JNC/Present
Av.	13	11	0.92
Stdev.	2	4	0.31
Max.	16	16	1.33
Min.	11	7	0.55

[From J. Takada, *J. Radiat. Res.*, **42**: Supple., S80 (2001)]

anisotropic radiation distribution, but also the validity of the second version of $D(r)$.

We should note that the values (14–26 mSv) for the seven persons calculated by the Countermeasures Head Office[3] were larger than the present and JNC evaluations. They evaluated individual doses within the 350-m zone without using any directional distribution of the radiation.

7.4.4   External Doses to 41 Houses West of the Accident Site

The directional distribution function of the radiation is clear only for the west side of the radiation source.[7] We do not know the directional distribution of the radiation to the east. Therefore, we focused on the 41 houses to the west within the 350-m zone. This number does not include the company with seven persons. The value of $\Phi(\theta_s)$, which is between 0.2 and 1.0 to the west is, remarkably, between 0.2 and 0.4 for the nearest residential area in the southwesterly direction, as shown in Fig. 7.4. The error of $\Phi(\theta_s)$ is 20% to 40% for $\Phi(\theta_s)$ between 0.2 and 1.0.

The number of houses in the westerly direction for which we evaluated the doses were 14 (18 in all directions), 19 (33) and 8 (19) within distance intervals of 95–200 m, 200–300 m and 300–350 m, respectively. The total numbers of people and buildings (including companies and shops) were 301 (141 residents) and 70 (43 houses), respectively, within the 350-m zone (Tokaimura local government data). The first dose evaluation for the public was carried out using eq. (7.2) with the first version of $D(r, t)$.[2,9] However, $D(r, t)$ was revised after making a big correction of dose for the burst at the initial period.[12] A good coincidence between D_i (JNC) and D_i (Present) using the second version of $D(r, t)$ supports the validity of the second revision. We therefore reevaluated the dose using the revised $D(r, t)$. Since the author does not know the site data for each resident, which were taken by Head Office of Countermeasures, the individual doses could not be evaluated in this study. We therefore estimated the doses at each house site. The effective dose for each house (j) was calculated using

$$D\ (r_j,\ \theta_j) = TF_j\Phi\ (\theta_j)\ D\ (r_j,\ 10\text{:}35\text{-}16\text{:}00) \tag{7.3}$$

where $D\ (r_j,\ 10\text{:}35\text{-}16\text{:}00)$ is the outdoor maximum dose at site j at distance r_j between 10:35 and 16:00. In this calculation, r_i and θ_j were determined for the actual sites of residents using a local map.[14] The time of 16:00 was the time of official evacuation of the 350-m zone.

The meaning of TF_s is the same as mentioned above. The structure and materials of the houses in this area were ordinary Japanese style. The value of TF_s for wooden houses, which was evaluated by the Head Office of Countermeasures, was 0.41–0.55 for neutrons and 0.54–0.69 for γ-rays.[3] The actual value for each site is probably less than these values due to the presence of furniture and clusters of homes in the residential areas near the JCO campus. In this study, we calculated the doses using two imaginary cases for shielding in the residential areas. One was an outdoor dose of $TF_s = 1.0$, which corresponds to the maximum dose at each site. The other was an indoor dose of $TF_s = 0.4$. The positive error from TF_s may be 37% for only the nearest houses.

The effective doses within the 350-m zone are summarized in Fig. 7.5. The average doses were estimated to be 0.7 and 1.7 mSv for indoors and outdoors, respectively, in this zone. The maximum values were 3.1 and 7.9 mSv for indoors and outdoors, respectively. We note that the house with the highest dose was not the nearest house, at a distance of 102 m to the southwest. This was due to the

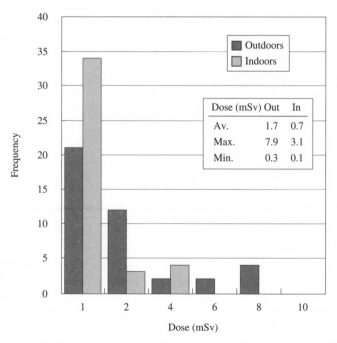

Fig. 7.5 Frequency distribution of the external effective doses to 41 houses within the 350-m zone. This does not include the site of the neighboring company with the seven persons described in the text.

[From J. Takada, *J. Radiat. Res.*, **42**: Supple., S81 (2001)] large shielding of the JCO campus. Most area residents were assumed to be indoors, except for some workers on September 30. In this case, 83% of the residents within the 350-m zone experienced external doses of less than 1 mSv. The total error of the indoor dose for the 41 houses is ± 46% to ± 67%.

The average doses within the 200-m zone were estimated to be 1.4 and 3.5 mSv for indoors and outdoors, respectively. The minimum values were 0.3 and 0.9 mSv for indoors and outdoors, respectively. This low-dose exposure in the nearest residential zone was due to the shielding by Building E and others, as shown in Fig. 7.4.

A radiological survey of the population within the 350-m zone on the day of the accident exhibited abnormal indications for only the seven persons discussed above, but not for those in the residential structures nearest the accident site. This suggests that the maximum dose for people within the 350-m zone was less than the does (11 mSv) of the above seven persons. Moreover, the survey showed a good qualitative coincidence with the present dose reconstruction based on the anisotropic radiation distribution. The maximum value of the doses for residents was estimated to be 3.1 mSv in this study.

On the other hand, the survey is inconsistent with the dose estimated by the Head Office of Countermeasures.[3] The estimated doses for the population within the 350-m zone were seven persons between 5 and 10 mSv, four persons between 10 and 15 mSv, and one person between 20 and 25 mSv. The maximum value was 21 mSv. The dose of five persons in their research was at the same level as that of the seven persons. Therefore, the results of the radiological survey on the population within the 350-m zone do not support the estimation by the Head Office of Countermeasures. This is because the anisotropic distribution of radiation was not taken into consideration in its report.

There is other direct evidence which supports a relatively low dose for the nearest residential area in the southwesterly direction. Kofuji et al. measured the radioactivity of phosphorus-32 (P-32) produced by the chlorine-35 (Cl-35) (n, α) P-32 reaction in table salt of houses.[15] The data showed a lower activity in the nearest residential area (within 200 m) compared with those in other directions.

7.5 Summary

A criticality accident occurred in a conversion facility of the uranium fuel processing factory of JCO Co., Ltd., in Tokaimura, Japan, on September 30, 1999. The nuclear reaction continued for 19 hours, resulting in fission of about 1 mg U-235. This nuclear accident was evaluated as level 4 on the International Nuclear Event Scale.

The nearest resident was only 100 m from the uranium source. The local government of Tokaimura intervened two hours after the beginning of the accident (H+2), deciding to order residents of the surrounding area to seek shelter elsewhere. Emergency evacuation of residents within a 350-m zone around the factory was carried out at H+5. Criticality was terminated at H+19 by draining the water from around the precipitation vessel where the accident occurred.

The thyroid dose received by the population around the accident site was estimated to be less than 0.1 mSv from the leakage of iodine radioactivity. The main exposure was due to neutrons and γ-rays from the uranium source. The nearest residential area in the southwesterly direction was shielded fairly well by the factory building. The present dose reconstruction for the 350-m zone to the west showed an average value of 0.7 mSv and a maximum value of 3.1 mSv as the indoor dose, assuming an effective transmittance of 0.4 for all houses. If all the residents within the 350-m zone were indoors during the accident, 83% of the houses might have received external doses of less than 1 mSv. However, seven workers in a neighboring company experienced doses of between 11 and 16 mSv.

Three workers of the JCO factory, who were manufacturing 18.8% enriched uranyl nitrate solution, suffered doses of between 1 and 20 GyEq. Two of them received doses more than 6 GyEq and died. Twenty-four persons who worked to terminate the criticality received a mean dose of 15 mSv with a maximum of less than 50 mSv.

Three members of the ambulance team aiding the exposed workers indicated external doses of between 5 and 9 mSv. Since they did not have personal dosimeters, doses were estimated by whole-body counting for Na-24. Some policemen who were assigned around JCO Company as the criticality continued, suffered doses over 1 mSv, the maximum being 4.9 mSv.

The total amount of uranium fissioned was about one milligram, or roughly one millionth that of the Hiroshima nuclear bomb. The amount of radioactivity leaked was relatively small and had negligible impact on the environment. The individual dose to the population was less than 16 mSv. Aside from the loss of life and as-yet unascertained long-term health effects the Tokaimura accident was a relatively minor disaster classified as level 4 on the International Nuclear Event Scale and left no long-term nuclear hazard in the area. Risk of late effects on the population must be negligibly small from the dose evaluation. However, the psychological impact on local society and all of Japan was considerable. It was responsible for an economic loss of over one hundred million U.S. dollars for the local community.

REFERENCES

1. Head Office for Emergency Countermeasures of the Criticality Accident in Tokaimura, *Conference documents of the 1st meeting on October 1, 1999* (1999) (in Japanese).
2. Head Office of Countermeasures in Science and Technology Agency of Japan (November 5, 1999), *Status of the Accident in JCO Tokai and Effects on the Environment*, No.66, 1-1, Document of the Atomic Energy Safety Committee (in Japanese).
3. Head Office of the Investigation for the Criticality Accident, Science and Technology Agency, (January 31, 2000), *Dosimetry Study for Residents around JCO Accidental Site and Future Work* (in Japanese).

4. T. Mitsugashira, M. Hara, T. Nakanishi, T. Sekine, R. Seki, S. Kojima, *J. Environmental. Radioactivity*, **50**, 21 (2000).
5. Head Office of Countermeasures in Science and Technology Agency of Japan (December 22, 1999), *Estimation of Radioactive Iodine Release and Dose in the JCO Criticality Accident, Dose Evaluation (Basic Data) around the JCO Tokai Accident*, No. 11-3-1 (in Japanese).
6. Nuclear Power Safety Committee, *White Paper on Nuclear Power*, Printing Bureau of the Ministry of Finance (2000) (in Japanese).
7. J. Takada, S. Suga, K. Kitagawa, M. Ishikawa, S. Takeoka, M. Hoshi, H. Watanabe, A. Itoho, N. Hayakawa, *J. Radiat. Res.*, **42**, 47 (2001).
8. J. Takada, *J. Radiat. Res.*, **42**: Suppl., S75 (2001).
9. J. Takada, M. Hoshi, *J. Environmental Radioactivity*, **50**, 43 (2000).
10. H. Mizuniwa, O. Kurihara, T. Yoshida, K. Isaki, T. Norio, T. Momose, H. Kobayashi, N. Hayashi, K. Miyabe, K. Noda, M. Kanamori, K. Shinohara, *J. of the Atomic Energy Society of Japan*, **43**, 56 (2001) (in Japanese).
11. T. Momose, N. Tsujimura, T. Tasaki, K. Kanai, O. Kurihara, N. Hayashi, K. Shinohara, *J. Radiat. Res.*, **42**, Suppl., S95 (2001).
12. Head Office of Countermeasures in Science and Technology Agency of Japan. No. 9-3 (December 11, 1999) *Reevaluation of Dosimetry around the JCO Accident* (in Japanese).
13. W.A. Woolson, M.L. Gritzner, S.D. Egbert, J.A. Robert, M.D. Otis, *House and Terrain Shielding, US-Japan Joint Reassessment of Atomic Bomb Radiation Dosimetry in Hiroshima and Nagasaki*, DS86, Radiation Effects Research Foundation, Vol.1, 227-305 (1987).
14. *Star Map Tokai Ibaraki*, Zenrin, Kita Kyushu (1999).
15. H. Kofuji, K. Komura, Y. Yamada, M. Yamamoto, *J. Environmental Radioactivity*, **50**, 49 (2000).

8

Nuclear Hazard and Recovery

In the previous chapter, individual nuclear disasters and hazards of various types were described. This chapter is a discussion on the concept of hazard in nuclear disaster, summarizing the present radiological status of hazards throughout the world as well as recovery. The final section is a review of the social recovery of Hiroshima after the bombing.

8.1 Concept of Nuclear Hazard

When considering a nuclear disaster from the viewpoint of protection, it is essential to understand the concept of nuclear hazard from the analysis of several nuclear disasters in the past. We can provide appropriate protection for the public against nuclear disasters by understanding the characteristics of the hazard.

The most remarkable characteristic in nuclear disasters is the short- and/or long-term radioactive pollution concerning neutron activations or fission products of plutonium (or uranium), etc. (Fig. 8.1). The nuclear hazard continues for some time but the radioactive level decreases with time by decay of radioactive nuclides and by some environmental mechanisms. This kind of hazard has its own recovery mechanisms. The half-life of the hazard depends on the kind of disaster. The shortest hazard is a neutron activation case such as ground zero after the Hiroshima bomb. The longest hazard is an underground nuclear explosion as found in weapons test sites or industrial applications.

The population living near the hazard suffers radiation exposure. Since various radioactive nuclides are involved in the hazard, risk to humans and environments varies. It is useful for protection against disasters to classify these various radioactive nuclides into three kinds of hazards from the viewpoint of half life or qualitative difference of influence.

The first is the short-term hazard during the month following the occurrence of disaster. The radioactive materials in this case are iodine, fission products (FP) with a short half-life and neutron-activated materials. These are the materials which cause heavy exposure to radiation by a population. In addition to acute radiation syndrome, they cause long-term health effects such as thyroid cancer, leukemia and other cancers.

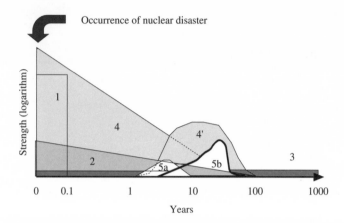

Fig. 8.1 Strength of effects on environment, human body and psychology due to nuclear hazard and its time sequences. 1: Short-term nuclear hazard which consists of short life fission products and neuron-induced radioactive materials, 2: Long-range hazard which consists of radioactive cesium and strontium, 3: Super long-term hazard which consists of plutonium and depleted uranium and others, 4: Occurrence and continuation of psychological effects, 5a: Health effect such as thyroid cancer or leukemia, 5b: Other cancers. There are a remarkable number of acute syndromes or death in the case of combat use of nuclear weapons.

In the case of Chernobyl, the worst accident in the history of nuclear facilities, the maximum dose to the public was level C due to this short-term hazard. The maximum dose for the thyroid was about 10 sieverts.[1,2] 80% of the thyroid dose was due to the intake of milk polluted with radioactive iodine.[2] The thyroid dose rate decreased substantially after one month. In the city of Pripyat where laborers at the nuclear power plant lived, iodine drugs were distributed for thyroid protection. They were not distributed in the other areas. Therefore, protection against this short-term hazard was indoor shelter, the non-intake of polluted milk, and intake of stable iodine. Even for an accident of level 7, these measures can be expected to provide sufficient radiation protection. Adequate protection in the first month after the nuclear hazard was not provided in the Chernobyl accident. Therefore, remarkable thyroid cancer occurred afterwards in a wide area.

The Three Mile Island accident in the United States was evaluated to be level 5, and the dose to the public was level E due to short-term hazard (less than 1mSv for whole body, 0.07 mSv for thyroid).[3,4] Therefore, in this accident, radiation protection was possible only by indoor sheltering. However, evacuation of pre-school children and expectant mothers within a 5-mile area was recommended two days after the occurrence of the accident. Tens of thousands of residents evacuated of their own will. The stable iodine drug which was prepared for use by 44,000 people for 10 days was not used.

The second hazard classification is long-term hazard due to environmental pollution by cesium-137 (Cs-137) (half-life: 30 y) and strontium-90 (Sr-90) (29 y). Since the former nuclide has a formation path through rare gas, it is easy to pollute distant areas. As for the latter, the pollution tends to be more limited to the disaster occurrence area than the former. The case of the Chernobyl nuclear reactor accident showed this aspect. However, in the case of a ground nuclear explosion, strontium causes a wide area of fallout. The Bikini nuclear disaster is an example. Strontium radioactivity pollution equal in level to that of cesium was found 170 km away.

The radioactivity in the environment does not always decay with the physical half-life. The effective half-life is usually shorter than the physical value locally. Indeed, the effective half-life of Cs-137 was about seven years on Rongelap Island. The annual dose for those living in the strict control zone (0.55 MBq/m) 10 years after the Chernobyl Accident is exposure of level D. It was level E below the 0.1 mSv for workers on Rongelap Island in 1999, 45 years after the fallout. These cases show that the risk of long-term hazard decreases gradually and becomes negligibly small. When the long-term hazard is at level D, most adults can tolerate the level, but children and women who may be pregnant require careful consideration. It is difficult to assert that there was not a problem for all those returning to Rongelap Island in 1957.[5]

Health effects which occur within 10 years after a nuclear incident are leukemia and thyroid cancer. The occurrence rate of the former was maximal five years after the bombing of Hiroshima and Nagasaki. The occurrence rate of the latter in children was maximal nine years after the Chernobyl accident.[6,7] Also, the occurrence rate of other cancers tended to increase little by little after 10 years in

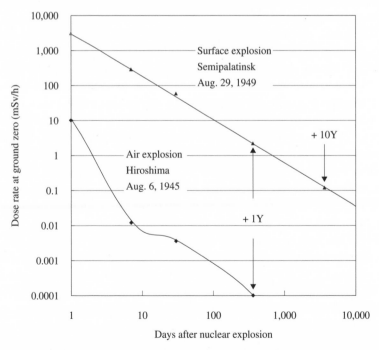

Fig. 8.2 Radiological decay at ground zero. Short-term nuclear hazard induced by neutron capture on the surface can be seen after the air explosion in Hiroshima. Long-term nuclear hazard is seen after surface nuclear explosions.

Hiroshima and Nagasaki. It should be understood that the origin of these health effects is not the low dose exposure of a long-term hazard but the high dose exposure of a short-term hazard.

The third classification of hazard involves α radiation emitters with a physical half-life of more than 20,000 years, e.g., plutonium and uranium. It affects ground zero and some fallout area after a surface nuclear explosion. The area of pollution is small compared with the other types of hazards. In the case of a surface explosion of a large-scale nuclear weapon, this third type of hazard occurs in wide areas like the Marshall Islands. Hazards of this kind are found in the case of nuclear reactor accidents of level 7. The 30-km zone around Chernobyl is this kind of hazard. We believe that the effective half-life of this hazard may be shorter than its physical half-life but this is still unclear.

8.2 Psychological Influence and Over-reaction in Society

The psychological impact first affects the victims of an accident and others in the general population mainly when acute radiation syndrome occurs due to the accident. Even if acute radiation syndrome does not occur in a population, misgivings about health in the future emerged with fragmentary information on late health effects in Hiroshima and Nagasaki. The possibility of late health effects, especially, have great psychological impact on the local population and society in general. Such a psychological influence lasts after the short-term hazard ends as well.

Sometimes, the psychological impact causes physical effects. Insufficient information on individual dose and radiation protection has sometimes made people and society miss directional decisions, resulting in suicide, disruption of pregnancy or economical damage due to rumors in some nuclear hazards. Nor is social discrimination rare for victims. There was cessation of social services by the administration, including mail, telephone and supply of electric power in the restricted zone after the Chernobyl accident. The psychological impact was considerable. In many cases, such events resulted in over-reaction on the part of society.

The Tokaimura criticality accident in Japan was evaluated as being of level 4 on the international nuclear event scale. However, the Chernobyl accident was level 7. Nuclear events equal to or less than level 3 are not even classified as accidents. The Tokaimura accident was small as a disaster. The public radiation exposure was level D at maximum. Moreover, 83% of the houses within a 350-m zone was level E. However, the damage due to rumor cost US$ 0.1 billion and the psychological impact on the residents and society was considerable. Secondary damage tends to generate more than the actual harm after a nuclear disaster.

The way the media report the disaster may also be a large factor. Of course, proper scientific information must be given out by the accident countermeasure headquarters. Moreover, unless the victims of an accident, reporters and other receivers of relevant information organize well to obtain knowledge concerning radiation protection on a daily basis, scientific and social communication will not work well in emergency situations.

8.3 Summary of Nuclear Disasters Worldwide

Nuclear disasters that occurred in the world since the mid 20th century have been related to combat use of nuclear weapons, their development, industrial use and accidents in nuclear fuel cycle and power plants. Some of them caused unacceptable radiation exposure to area residents and radioactive contamination of the environment.

From the viewpoint of scale of radiation source in our research, the largest and smallest ware the US thermonuclear explosion in Bikini Atoll (a thousand times larger than the Hiroshima N-bomb) and the Tokaimura criticality accident (one millionth that of the Hiroshima N-bomb), respectively. From the viewpoint of scale of distance between the source of disaster and affected residential area, the shortest and longest were Tokaimura (100 m) and Zaborie (220 km), respectively.

Concerning to the dose level on residents at the time of disaster, the highest were the fatal levels in Hiroshima and Nagasaki, and the smallest was the medical examination level in Tokaimura. The people of Rongelap Island would have suffered fatal doses if they had not been evacuated two days after the beginning of radioactive fallout.

All the hazards investigated by the author have been classified into six

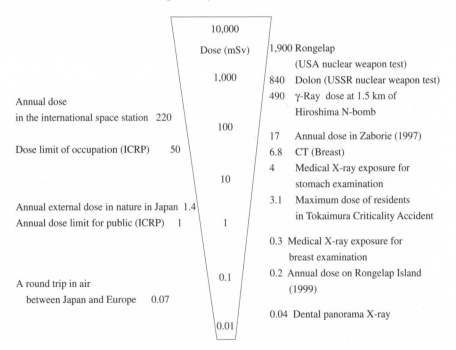

Fig.8.3 Comparison of radioactive doses in nuclear hazards and other situations.

Table 8.1 Summary of the main nuclear hazards in the world

Nuclear disaster area		Exposure year	Exposure level	Radiation sources	Scale of radiation source	Distance from source (km)	Exposure path	Radiation level in 2000
Hiroshima	Japan	1945	A	Combat use of nuclear weapon	15 kt	0.6	Direct	F
Dolon	Kazakhstan	1949	B	Nuclear weapon tests	18 Mt	50	FO	F
Musulyumovo	Russia	1949	B	Nuclear waste pollution	100 PBq	78	River	E
Rongelap	Marshall Islands	1954	A⁻	Nuclear weapon tests	15 Mt	175	FO	E
Zaborie	Russia	1986	C	Nuclear reactor accident	2 EBq	220	FO	D
Tokaimura	Japan	1999	D	Criticality accident	1 mg of U-235	0.1	Direct	F

The distance for Dolon is the distance between Dolon and the test site boundary.
FO: Fallout
Dose level:

A Fatal dose $\geqq 4$ Gy   D Medical examination $\leqq 10$ mGy
B Acute and late effects   1-3 Gy   E Less than 1 mGy a year
C Late effects, effects to fetus 0.1-1 Gy   F Effects due to nuclear disaster can be ignored

categories, A through F, by dose, as seen Table 8.1. All the dose levels for the year 2000 were level D or less. There is low-level contamination or less than detectable limit of residual radioactivity except in a few residential areas like Zaborie.

8.4 Radiological Status of Nuclear Hazards in the World

The *in-situ* investigations were conducted by the author between 1995 and 2000. Except for Tokaimura, the investigations were carried out more than ten years after the occurrence of the disaster. The elapsed time till measurement was about 10 years for the Chernobyl accident and more than 40 years for the Mayak pollution, Bikini test, Hiroshima nuclear bomb and Semipalatinsk tests (for Dolon). In the long term, attenuation of nuclear contamination in the local environment was noted. The Tokaimura accident was the exception with no remarkable radioactive contamination.

These nuclear hazards, at sites far from each other, are physically independent occurrences. The natural environment differs considerably among them. For example, Rongelap, which suffered fallout from the Bikini thermonuclear explosion, is a small atoll of only two meters sea level in the southern Pacific Ocean. Zaborie, which suffered fallout from the Chernobyl accident, is agricultural land far inland. Sakha, where underground nuclear explosions were conducted, is located in perpetually frozen land. Therefore, migration or diffusion of radioactive materials on the earth's surface was quite different, reflecting the various environments and weather patterns.

Cs-137, Sr-90 and Pu (plutonium) are remarkable nuclides that can cause long-term residual contamination, with a half-life of about 30 years for the former two and 24,000 years for Pu-239. The contamination densities for these three nuclides on land surface are plotted in Fig. 8.4. This is a world map showing the densities of the remaining three kinds of radioactivity as the axis. The pollution density of cesium and strontium is shown by the horizontal and vertical axes of the graph. The pollution by plutonium is shown by the radius. The value represents the radioactivity of plutonium for each circle.

Some values are unknown for some hazards. The strontium data for Dolon, which is unknown, is plotted at the bottom of the figure. Data from ground material in 1978 reported by Robinson[12] have been added for the islands in the Rongelap Atoll.

The severest nuclear hazard areas are located in the upper right part or large circle in this figure. Chernobyl's strict control zone Zaborie and the northern islands of Rongelap Atoll are found here. Although the flood plane of the Techa River is most contaminated by Sr-90 and Cs-137, no one lives there. The residents of Muslyumovo near the river have not drunk river water since 1961.

On the other hand, the no remarkable or low contamination areas are located in the lower left part of the figure, e.g., Dolon, Muslyumovo and Rongelap. The levels in Hiroshima and Nagasaki are equal to or less than the levels in this area.

There are two remarkable areas concerning the ratio between Sr-90 and Cs-

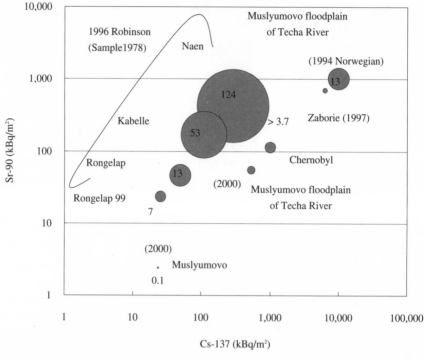

Fig. 8.4 Long-term nuclear hazards map with 3D axis including surface densities of Cs-137, Sr-90 and Pu-239, -240. The density of plutonium (kBq/m²) is proportional to the radius of the circle. Reference data for Muslyumovo,[10] three islands of Naen, Kabelle, Rongelap in 1996,[12] 30-km zone in Chernobyl,[9] Dolon.[14]

137. Rongelap Atoll is about 1:1 and other areas are 1:10. The reason for this is unknown.

The main source of external radiation was Cs-137 and natural nuclides in 1995-2000. Here we summarize the dose rate in the environment in a graph with the dose rate on the Y axis and Cs-137 pollution on the X axis.

γ-Ray dose rate is proportional to Cs-137 density on the ground surface in highly contaminated areas. However, the dose rate is not proportional to the Cs-137 density in low contamination areas where the radiation of natural sources is dominant. Thus the dominant radiation in Dolon, Hiroshima and Teya comes from natural sources with low contamination by Cs-137.

Areas with severe external exposure are located towards the upper right in Fig. 8.5. The safe areas are located towards the lower left. The most severe area of external exposure in the figure is Masani within 10 km of Chernobyl. Two scientists investigated the environment over one year, alternating two-week stays. The second area is Zaborie, where some residents continue to live of their own free will. The third is Hoiniki in the nonrestricted zone, where people with children live. We know that victims of thyroid cancer reside in this area.

The next group of residential areas show remarkable Cs-137 contamination but low dose rates in the environment. Bashakl, Muslyumobo and Rongelap are in

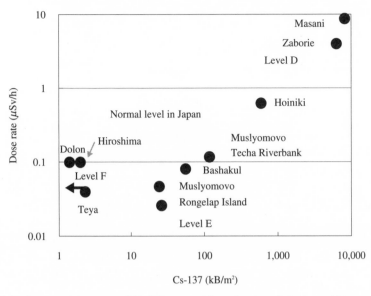

Fig. 8.5 Environmental dose rate and Cs-137 measured in nuclear hazards in the world between 1995 and 2000.

this group. Radiation in this area is equal or lower than the natural background level of Japan or Kazakhstan. The former two villages have residents. Rongelap has had no residents since 1985. However, workers have been staying on the island for the construction of a resettlement program since 1998.

8.5 Body Burden of Radioactivity for Residents in Nuclear Hazard Areas

Residents who live in nuclear hazard areas intake radioactive materials through inhalation, food or water. Cs-137 body burden is plotted against Cs-137 contamination on the surface of land. Fig. 8.6 shows data for four areas. The area shown without data in this figure has less than the detectable limit of contamination. Since the biological half-life of cesium is about 100 days, this nuclide comes from current contamination.

The highest body burden of Cs-137 in our investigation was found in Zaborie. The value of Cs-137 was 1.5 kBq/kg resulting in an annual internal dose of 3 mSv in 1997.

Mushroom is a major food source of body contamination. Mushroom sampled in Masani, where the contamination was higher than in Zaborie, showed Cs-137 of 33 kBq/kg. However, scientists staying there did not eat the local food in Masani.

The number of cases of measurements for Sr-90 and Pu is smaller than that for Cs-137. The reason is that transmittance of β- or α-rays from the former nuclides is much lower than γ-rays from the latter, i.e., it is very difficult to measure Sr-90 or Pu from body surface. However, successful β-ray measurement using the author's portable laboratory was conducted on the front teeth for Sr-90

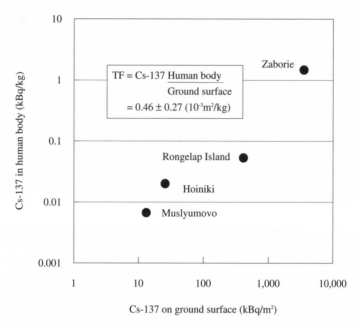

Fig. 8.6 Cs-137 body burden of residents living in nuclear hazard areas in the world.

among the residents of Muslyumovo.

A remarkably high body burden of Sr-90 was observed among residents upstream and midstream of the Techa River. It is believed to be the highest in the world. Degteva[13] reports that the Sr-90 content in the population is decreasing gradually since 1952, but it is still an average of 4 kBq (about 67 Bq/kg) in whole body. More than half the 14,500 permanent residents along the Techa have red bone marrow doses between 0.1 and 0.5 Gy.

Shevchuk reported about 100 Bq Sr-90 body burden in 1993 for the area contaminated by Chernobyl in Belarus.[15] According to a pollution map for 1992, Sr-90 density in the 30-km zone of Belarus was equal to or more than 111 kBq/m².[16]

8.6 Decay of Local Radioactive Contamination Due to Environmental Factors

Residents of Dolon suffered radiation exposure of level B from radioactive fallout due to surface nuclear explosion in the testing period. However, there is no remarkable residual radioactivity in the village after 50 years. Since the half-life of Cs-137 is 30 years, the present radiological state connot be explained only by physical decay. If the rapid diffusion of nuclear pollution occurred in the horizontal direction, this phenomenon is understandable. The reason may be the dry climate of Kazakhstan.

The surface radioactive contamination of Rongelap Island with a maximum sea level of only about two meters may have been swept away by the action of waves. The land there consists of coral sand. Carbonic acid calcium, the main material, belongs to the same chemical family as strontium. From the depth profile analysis, we noted that 90% of Cs-137 and plutonium was stored 15 cm deep from the surface. On the other hand, Sr-90 diffuses deeply; the density at 30 cm was almost the same as at the surface. Therefore, the amount of Cs-137 and plutonium near the surface was reduced by the washing of the waves. However, strontium in the deep layer was not swept out by ocean waves. This may be the reason for the higher ratio of strontium than cesium on Rongelap Island than noted in other sites.

The radioactivity on the surface contaminated by fallout is decreased not only by physical decay but also by environmental factors. For example, if Cs-137 decays 50% by nuclear decay and another 50% by an environmental factor, it decreases by a total of 25%. Radiological recovery around the Semipalatinsk Test Site and Rongelap Island may be cases involving large environmental factors.

In contrast, horizontal diffusion of radioactivity may be relatively small in grassland and forests of the hinterland. Some artificial diffusion may occur by the transport of agricultural products or wood. Moreover, there is decontamination measure for this.

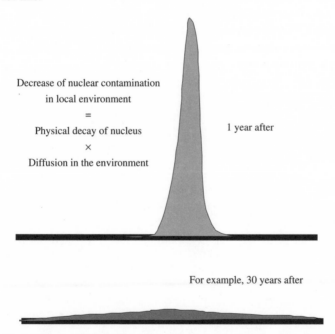

Decrease of nuclear contamination
in local environment
=
Physical decay of nucleus
×
Diffusion in the environment

1 year after

For example, 30 years after

Fig. 8.7 Schematic illustration of decay of radioactivity in nuclear hazard areas.

8.7 Revival of Hiroshima

Hiroshima, the first city to suffer nuclear disaster, was destroyed on August 6, 1945, by a US nuclear weapon with a TNT equivalent of 15 kt. By December of that year, 140,000 victims had died. They suffered late health effects of leukemia and other cancers and experienced physical and mental difficulties which are difficult to imagine. The survivors worked steadily for the revival of Hiroshima without deserting the land.

Radiation measurements at ground zero were carried out by a group under Dr. Bunsaku Arakatsu of Kyoto University on August 10 or by a group led by Dr. Yukio Miyazaki of RIKEN, the Institute of Physical and Chemical Research, on October 1. The measurements showed rapid decrease of activity.[17]

Temporary housing began to be built in October.[18] The main railway of the city was restored, lifting the citizens' spirits. On November 18, Ebisu Shrine was reconstructed on a burned field in the central part of the city. Ebisu Festival and a revival meeting took place the next day.

The Hiroshima revival bureau was established on January 8, 1946. In April, Hiroshima's revival city plan was established and a five-year plan was set up. The supply of city gas was resumed in the same month. On May 31, the water supply was restored to 70% of the city. The population grew to 150,000 that year. Although physicists forecast that the vegetation would not grow for 70 years, weeds put out buds the following summer. Many vegetable gardens were cultivated due to serious food shortage.

The Peace Commemoration City Construction Law, which aimed to rebuild a city symbolizing permanent peace, was legislated in 1949 and became the basis for reviving fiscal resources.

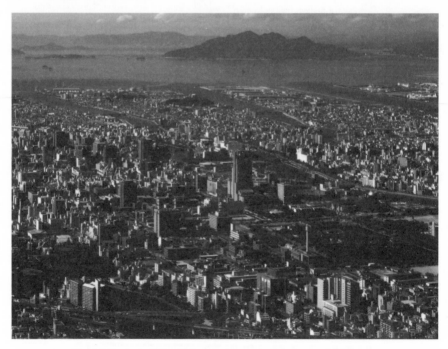

Fig. 8.8 Revival of Hiroshima. Ground zero is at the center of the figure.
[©Chugoku Shimbun, Japan (1994)]

The citizens of Hiroshima achieved remarkable recovery and succeeded in the reconstruction of a beautiful city. The population exceeded one million in 2000. The radiation at ground zero was less than 0.1 μSv/h in 2000, a normal value found throughout all of Japan.

REFERENCES

1. L.A. Ilyn, *Chernobyl: Myth and Reality*, Megapolis, Moscow (1995).
2. S. Shinkarev, *private communication*.
3. *Nuclear Regulatory Commission Conference Documents*, May 3, USA (1979).
4. *Nuclear Regulatory Commission Preliminary Notification*, PNO-79-67 A-Z, April-June (1979).
5. J. Takada, M. Yamamoto, *Dosimetry Study in Rongelap Island 1999, KEK Proceedings*, 2001-14 (2001).
6. I. Shigematsu, C. Itoh, N. Kamada, M. Akiyama, H. Sasaki, eds., *Effects of A-bomb Radiation on the Human Body*, Harwood Academic Publishers and Bunkodo Co., Ltd. Tokyo (1995).
7. E.P. Demidchik, Yu.E. Demidchik, Z.E. Gedrevich, A.G. Mrochek, V.A. Ostapenko, J.E. Kenigsberg, E.E. Buglova, Yu.D. Sidorov, V.A. Kondratovich, V.V. Baryach, E.P. Dubouskaya, V.M. Veremeichyk, S.V. Mankouskaya, *Thyroid Cancer in Belarus, Chernobyl Message for the 21st Century*, pp.69-75, Elsevier (2002).
8. H. Yasuda, *Radiation Science*, **40**, 159 (1997) (in Japanese).
9. The International Chernobyl Project, *Surface Contamination Maps*, IAEA (1991).
10. Joint Norwegian-Russian Expert Group for Investigation of Radioactive Contamination in the Northern Areas, *Sources Contributing to Radioactive Contamination of the Techa River and Areas surrounding the Mayak Production Association, Urals, Russia* (1997).
11. A.V. Akleyev, M.F. Kisselyov, ed., *Medical-biological and Ecological Impacts of Radioactive Contamination of the Techa River*, Russian Federation Health Ministry, Federal Office of Medical-Biological Issues and Emergencies, Urals Research Center for Radiation Medicine, Moscow (2000).
12. W.L. Robinson, V.E. Noshkin, C.L. Conrado, R.J. Eagle, J.L. Brunk, T.A. Jokela, M.E. Mount, W.A. Phillips, A.C. Stoker, M.L. Stuart, K.M. Wong, *Health Phys.*, **73**, 37 (1997).
13. M.O. Degteva, V.P. Kozhenrov, E.I. Tolstykh, *Radiat. Prot. Dosimetry*, **79**, 155 (1998).
14. M. Yamamoto, M. Hoshi, J. Takada, A. Sekerbaev, B. Gusev, *J. Radio Analytical and Nuclear Chemistry*, **242**, 63 (1999).
15. V.E. Shevchuk, *private communication*.
16. Committee of Geodesy of the Council of the Ministry of the Republic of Byelorussia, *Map of the Radioactrve Situation in the Territory of the Republic of Belarus in Accordance with Data in January 1992*, West Air-Geodesy Enterprise, Minsk (1992).
17. Science Council of Japan, Reports on the atomic bomb disaster investigation (1953) (in Japanese).
18. *Chugoku Shimbun*, Records of Hiroshima (1995).

Appendices

A1 Glossary

Energy: Ability to do work. Includes heat energy, excercise energy, position energy and others. Measured in physical units of joules or electron volts.

Electron volt (eV): 1 eV is the value of energy of one electron in an electric field at 1 volt voltage. This energy unit is often used to represent energy of atoms, nuclei and radiation. For example, the energy of the γ-rays from cesium-137 (Cs-137) is 660 keV. The energy of visible light is about 2 eV.

Absorbed dose: This is the energy absorbed per unit mass and is measured in units of joules per kilogram, which is given the special name gray (Gy).

Dose equivalent: Radiation quantity used for radiation protection purposes that expresses dose on a common scale for all radiations. The unit is the sievert (Sv).

Dose equivalent = Quality factor of radiation · Absorbed dose · Correction factor

The quality factor is the value which depends on the radiation and the energy. As the factor, one is used for γ-rays and electrons (β-rays), ten is used for neutrons (when the energy distribution is unclear), twenty is used for α particles. The correction factor is a value near 1.

Effective dose: This is the sum of the weighted equivalent doses in all tissues and organs of the body. The unit is the sievert (Sv). It is given by the expression

$$E = \sum_{T} w_T \cdot H_T$$

where H_T is the equivalent dose in tissue or organ T and w_T is the weighing factor for tissue T.

Radioactivity: Rate of decay or disintegration of radioactive material. One decay per one second is 1 becquerel (Bq). Total radioactivity of potassium -40 and carbon -14 for the adult in Japan as the crude radioactivity in the body is about 7000 Bq.

Half-life: Time in which half the nuclei of a given radioisotope disintegrates. This is the physical half-life. Biological half-life is the time in which a biological system eliminates by natural processes half the amount of a foreign substance that has entered. See A4.

Table A.1 Units of some radiation quantities

Quantity	SI unit	Symbol
Activity	Becquerel	Bq
Absorbed dose	Gray	Gy
Dose equivalent	Sievert	Sv

A2 Dose Level and Risk of Radiation Exposure

It is easy to understand the risk from radiation exposure of an accident and disaster radiation exposure when based on a dose of 1 Sv because acute radiation sickness occurs at levels over 1 Sv. Since most people are not familiar with the Sievert, detailed dose values using this unit are not clear to them. Therefore, the author has proposed six levels classification of dose with threshold values. These range from the most dangerous level A to level F, at which level the effects of a nuclear disaster can be ignored. The threshold values have been recognized from studies by many scientists and the ICRP. These are 4, 1, 0.1, 0.01 and 0.001 Sv.

Table A.2 Dose level and risk of radiation exposure

Dose level	Risk	Dose* (Sv)
A	lethality	≥ 4
B	acute syndrome, late disease	≥ 1
C	effects on fetus, late disease	≥ 0.1
D	somewhat safe	≤ 0.01
E	safe	≤ 0.001
F	negligible	

*Dose for whole body
$0.1 < D^* < 0.1$
Basic information is summarized in appendices A1, 5 and 6 for a clearer understanding of the category of dose level with some risk.

A3 Metric Multiples and Submultiples

Designations of multiples and subdivisions of any unit may be arrived at by combining with the name of the unit.

Table A.3 Metric multiples and submultiples

Symbol	Meaning	
E (exa)	10^{18}	
P (peta)	10^{15}	
T (tera)	10^{12}	
G (giga)	10^9	billion
M (mega)	10^6	million
k (kilo)	10^3	thousand
c (centi)	10^{-2}	
m (milli)	10^{-3}	
μ (micro)	10^{-6}	
n (nano)	10^{-9}	
p (pico)	10^{-12}	

A4 External and Internal Exposure from Radioactivity

External exposure is exposure in which the human body is irradiated by external radio nuclides. Examples include exposure from the fireball of a nuclear explosion or from neutron-induced radionuclides and long-term nuclear hazards.

Internal exposure is exposure in which the human body intakes radio-nuclides. The routes are intake of contaminated food and water, inhalation of radioactive dust and gas, and absorption through skin. Each radionuclide is deposited in different tissue depending on the element. The biological half-life of a nuclide is completely different from its physical half-life.

Table A.4 Neutron-induced nuclides

Nuclide	$T_{1/2}$
Al-28	2.2 m
Mn-56	2.6 h
Na-24	15 h
Fe-56	44 d
Sc-46	83 d

Table A.5 Health effects due to internal exposure by some radioactive nuclides

Nuclides	Physical half-life	Biological half-life	Deposition organs	Internal activity of 1mSv exposure equivalent*	Main effects
Cs-137	30 y	100 d	Muscles, Whole-body	77 kBq	Leukemia, sterility
Sr-90	29 y		Bones, teeth	36 kBq	Bone tumors, leukemia
I-131	8 d	80 d	Thyroid	45 kBq	Thyroid cancer, hypothyroidism
Pu-239	24,000 y	100 y (bones)	Bones, lungs, liver	4 kBq	Bone tumors, liver cancer
		40 y (liver)			Leukemia , lung cancer

*These values are calculated from effective dose coefficients for ingested particulates table B.1 of ICRP Publication 68. The dose corresponds to internal exposure for 50 years after ingestion of the radionuclide. In fact, since the physical half-life and the biological half life of Cs and I are relatively short, they will disappear rapidly from the body after ingestion.

A5 Radiation Effects on Human Body

Radiation diseases due to external exposure have been well studied on survivors of Hiroshima and Nagasaki. The disease is classified into acute effects and late effects with an incubation period of more than several years.

Tissues in which the frequency of cell splitting is high or the number of cell splitting is large, or the form and features of cells are nondifferentiated are radiation-sensitive. Bone marrow, small intestine, skin, the lens and gonads are especially sensitive to radiation. Fetuses and infants are radiation-sensitive as a whole.

Table A.6 Acute radiation disease due to whole-body exposure

Dose (mSv)	Symptom
$\leqq 250$	Almost no clinical symptom
500	Temporary decrease in lymphocytes
1,000	Vomiting, exhaustion, remarkable decrease in lymphocytes
1,500	Radiation intoxication in half the population
2,000	Long-term leukopenia
3,000	Temporary epilation
4,000	Death in half the population in 30 days

[Reproduced with permission from K. Watari, J. Inaba, *Radioactivity and the Human Body* (in Japanese), p.26, Kenseisha (1999)]

Table A.7 Threshold for deterministic effects

Effect	Threshold (mSv)
Temporary sterility	
Male (gland)	150
Female (ovary)	$\geqq 650$
Permanent sterility	
Male (gland)	$\geqq 3,500$
Female (ovary)	$\geqq 2,500$
Temporary epilation	3,000
Cataracts	2,000
Fetus	
Abortion (fertilization 0-15 days)	100
Malformation (fertilization 2-8 weeks)	100
Mental retardation (fertilization 8-15weeks)	120

[Reproduced with permission from Japan Health Physics Society ed., *New Radiation Effects on Human Body* (in Japanese), p.33, 37, 39, Maruzen (1993)]

A6 Recommendations of the International Commission on Radiological Protection and Related Values

The International Commission on Radiological Protection (ICRP) has reported recommendations to assist regulatory and advisory agencies at national, regional and international levels, mainly by providing guidance on the fundamental principles on which appropriate radiological protection can be based.

Table A.8 Recommended dose limits[*1]

Application	Dose limit	
	Occupational	Public
Effective dose	20 mSv per year, averaged over defined periods of 5 years[*2]	1 mSv per year[*3]
Annual equivalent dose in lens of the eye	150 mSv	15 mSv
skin	500 mSv	50 mSv
hands and feet	500 mSv	–

[*1]These dose limits apply to the sum of external and internal exposures.
[*2]The effective dose should not exceed 50 mSv in any single year. Additional restrictions apply to the occupational exposure of pregnant women.
[*3]In special cases, the average dose over 5 years does not exceed 1 mSv per year.
[Reproduced with permission from Intenational Commission on Radiological Production ed., *ICRP Publication*, p.60, Pergamon Press (1991) ©Elsevier Science]

Table A.9 Nominal probability coefficients for stochastic effects

Exposed population	Detriment ($10^{-2}Sv^{-1}$)			
	Fatal cancer	Nonfatal cancer	Severe hereditary effects	Total
Adult workers	4.0	0.8	0.8	5.6
Whole population	5.0	1.0	1.3	7.3

[Reproduced with permission from Intenational Commission on Radiological Production ed., *ICRP Publication*, p.60, Pergamon Press (1991) ©Elsevier Science]

A7 Radiation Shield

γ-Rays (photons), β-rays (electrons), α-rays (helium) and neutrons are given off as ionizing radiation from radioactive material. α-Rays can not penetrate several centimeters in air due to collisions with molecules of oxygen or nitrogen. α-Rays can be shielded by paper. β-Rays can be shielded by a metallic plate or a thick

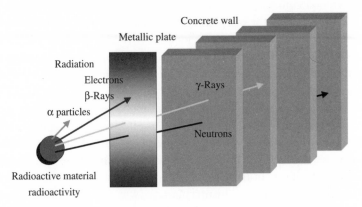

Fig. A.1 Shield against radiation.

cloth. Therefore, the interior of automobiles or houses is well shielded against α- and β-rays in a nuclear disaster. γ-Rays and neutrons can penetrate the walls of houses or buildings, but some offer shielding. Underground rooms are well shielded and safe.

Table A.10 Fallout γ-ray dose transmission factors
for various structures

Structure	Dose transmission factor
1 m underground	0.0002
Wooden house	0.3–0.6
Basement	0.05–0.1
Multistory building	
Upper stories	0.01
Lower stories	0.1

[From S. Glasstone, P.J. Dolan, *The Effects of Nuclear Weapons*, p.441, US Department of Defense (1977)]

A8 Radiation Protection in Emergencies

Effective countermeasures for public radiation protection in the case of a large-scale nuclear accident or nuclear explosion on the ground are introduced in this section. Those downwind from the site will suffer from the effects of a radioactive cloud (see Chapters 3, 4, 6). They will first suffer external γ radiation for whole body and β irradiation on the skin, and inhalation of radioactive materials outdoors. Several days later they will undergo internal exposure from food.

The first countermeasure is shelter during the emergency period. The building should be well enclosed to avoid penetration of radioactive gas or dusts. The home might be the best place with food, bed and other necessities, as well as from the psychological point of view. Basements and multistory buildings are much better than wooden houses for radiation shield (see A7) since they reduce external radiation exposure and inhalation of radionuclides and offer protection from β-burn on skin in the short term (see Chapter 8).

The second countermeasure is not to intake contaminated food or water, especially in the case of a short-term nuclear hazard with a high dose rate. The consumption of milk contaminated by iodine-131 (I-131) involves risk for thyroid cancer. In the Chernobyl accident 80% of thyroid dose originated from contaminated milk. Therefore, milk consumption should be stopped for about one month in a short-term nuclear hazard.

For preventive thyroid protection the intake of a reasonable amount of stable iodine 3 or 4 hours before inhalation of I-131 is effective. The amount is 100 mg a day for adults. This cuts off 95% of the dose of radioactive iodine to the thyroid. Iodine potassium tablets are prepared for the population living around a nuclear power plant. However, in the case of a major nuclear accident, the number of stable iodine tablets may be insufficient, as was the case in the Chernobyl accident. Japanese often eat seaweed, which is abundant in stable iodine. They usually store dried kelp in the home. This will be useful for thyroid protection in Japan.

If heavy radioactive fallout happens, residents should evacuate the contaminated area during or after the emergency period. One must be careful to protect against β irradiation and inhalation during the emergency. A mask over the mouth is recommended, and skin should not be exposed.

Evacuation some years after an emergency has occurred is open to question.

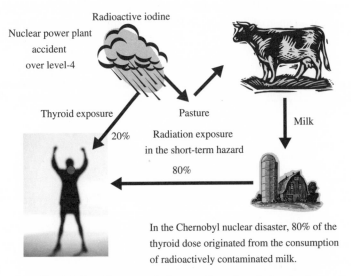

Fig. A.2 Thyroid exposure in the case of a nuclear plant accident.

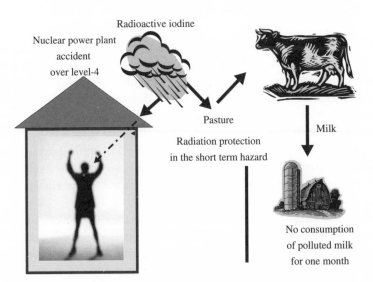

Fig. A.3 Radiation protection in the case of a nuclear plant accident.

There may only be a psychological effect, especially for adults. Decision making should be based on scientific information.

A9 Effects and Radiation Protection in the Case of Nuclear Weapons Terrorism

Small portable nuclear weapons have been developed in the USA and former USSR. The existence of the portable-type nuclear weapon became clear in 1997. It said that 84 portable nuclear weapons from Russia are missing. The US developed a small nuclear weapon of 28 kg in the 1960s and deployed it until 1989.

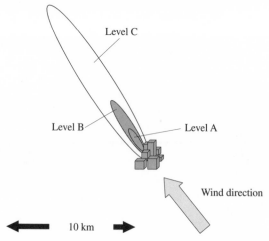

Fig. A.4 Simulation of radiation exposure by terrorism resulting from a nuclear weapon with a TNT equivalent of 1 kt.
[From J. Takada, *J. Hiroshima Med.*, **57**, 369 (2004)]

Let us consider terrorism with a nuclear weapon the equivalent of 1 kt of TNT in a city. The explosion produces a fireball with a diameter of 70 m and several million degrees centigrade, emitting thermal radiation, γ-rays, neutrons and shock wave. Estimating from the nuclear disaster in Hiroshima, an 800-m zone will be enormously affected by the shock wave and a 500-m zone will possibly be burned. However, in a city with many concrete buildings the blast and heat rays are somewhat blocked. People within an 800-m zone will suffer Level-A external dose by direct radiation from the fireball if there is no radiation shielding. Most people in buildings or basements will survive as was the case in Hiroshima where 78 individuals survived (see Chapter 1).

The most dangerous radiation source will be fission products and neutron-induced radioactive materials. In the case of the nuclear bombing occurring in a building in a city, a large amount of radioactive dust forms and covers the area downwind. The best way to protect oneself against radioactive dust is sheltering for more than 1 hour then evacuation by subway. Running away in the streets immediately after a bombing is extremely dangerous due to highly radioactive

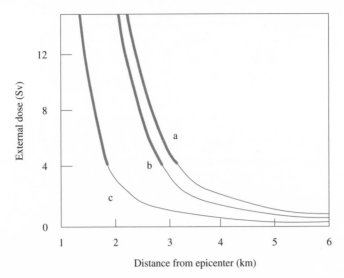

Fig. A.5 Dose as a function of distance from the epicenter for three different ways of evacuation. a: running away above ground for 1 hour, b: running for 15 minutes and then evacuating by subway, c: the best way, sheltering more than 1 hour and evacuating by subway (with 15 minutes running above ground).
[From J. Takada, *J. Hiroshima Med.*, **57**, 370 (2004)]

dust with a short half-life. The level of short half-life radionuclides decreases sharply during the period of sheltering. A mask to avoid inhalation of radioactive dust and glasses or goggles to protect the eyes against β-rays are recommended.

A10   Nuclear Fuel Recycling

After the production of thermal energy from uranium fuel at a nuclear power plant, fuel assemblies are taken out as spent fuel. This is reprocessed to extract residual uranium as well as plutonium which has been produced during irradiation in order to use them once more to feed the nuclear power plant. This is nuclear fuel recycling. Using the fuel mixture of plutonium oxide and uranium oxide in a light-water reactor raises the efficiency of uranium resources. The nuclear fuel recycling system with the fast breeder reactor may be the most promising energy system for the next thousand years throughout the world. A safe recycling system with final disposal technology should be developed to achieve this. This is a great challenge for the human race.

Uranium fuel for light-water reactors contains 2–4% of fissionable uranium, U-235. The rest is nonfissionable uranium, uranium-238 (U-238). There remains still about 1% of U-235 in spent fuel after 3–4 years of service in a reactor. One percent represents a substantial quantity, compared with the initial quantity which is 2–4%. The nonfissionable U-238 does not release any energy, but it can absorb neutrons to transform it into plutonium-239 (Pu-239), which is fissionable.

The use of plutonium permits more effective exploitation of uranium

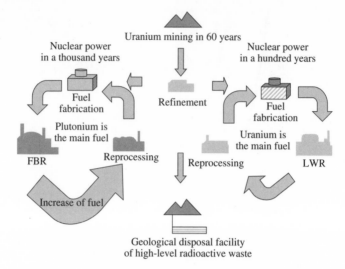

Fig. A.6 Nuclear fuel recycling.

resources. Plutonium can feed not only the thermal reactor when mixed with uranium to fabricate mixed fuel (MOX), but also the fast breeder reactor, which is expected to be the leading reactor in the future. Reprocessing is the operation to extract residual uranium and produce plutonium from spent fuel. The MOX fuel has been used over the past 30 years mainly in European countries such as France, Germany, Switzerland and Belgium, since the first loading of the BR-3 thermal reactor in Belgium in 1963. MOX fuel in thermal reactors was used in more than 3500 assemblies in the year 2000. Six fast breeder reactors (including one maintaining FBR) are operating in the world in 2003. Two are under construction in two countries and one FBR is under design in 2003.

The final disposal of high-level radioactive waste is the most important task in nuclear fuel recycling. There are two types. One is spent fuel and the other is vitrified waste. Glass of high-level radioactive waste which consists of nuclear fission products is solidized in a metallic container in the latter type. Both types of waste will be stored deep underground according to the disposal program of each country.

Table A.11 Reprocessing plants in the world (2003)

Country	Name	Installer	Location	Reprocessing capacity (t-Upr/year)		Start of operation
U.K.	B-205 Plant	British Nuclear Fuels Limited	Sellafield	Natural uranium	1500	1964
	B-204 Plant	〃	〃	Enriched uranium	400	1969
	THORP Plant	〃	〃	Enriched uranium	1200	1994
France	UP-1 Plant	Companie Générale des Matières Nucléaires	Marcoule	Natural uranium	400	1958
	UP-2 Plant	〃	La Hague	Enriched uranium	800	1994
	UP-3 Plant	〃	〃	Enriched uranium	800	1990
Japan	Tokai Plant	Japan Nuclear Cycle Development Institute	Tokaimura, Ibaraki Pref.	Enriched uranium	0.7t-Upr/day	1981
	Rokkasho Plant	Japan Nuclear Fuel Limited	Rokkashomura, Aomori Pref.	Enriched uranium	800	2006 (planned)
Russia	RT-1	Dept. of Nuclear Energy	Cheryabinsk	Enriched uranium	400	1977
India	Tronbay Plant	Baber Atomic Energy Center	Tronbay		30	1964
	Taraboul Plant	〃	Taraboul			
	Kalbacam	〃	Kalbacam		100	1998
Italy	Saluggia	ENAE				1983

Operating Plants in 2003 from ATOMICA (in Japanese)

Table A.12 Fast breeder reactors in the world (2003)

Reactor		Country	Output (MW) Thermal	Output (MW) Electric	Type of core[2]	First criticality	Present condition
Experimental reactor	FBTR	India	42.5	15	Loop	1985	Operating
	Joyo	Japan	140	–	Loop	1977[1]	Operating
	BOR-60	Russia	55	12	Loop	1968	Operating
	CEFR	China	65.5	25	Tank	(2005)	Under construction
Prototype reactor	Phenix	France	563	250	Tank	1973	Operating
	PFBR	India	1,250	500	Tank	(2009)	Design stage
	Monju	Japan	714	280	Loop	1994	Under maintenance
Demonstration reactor	BN-600	Russia	1,470	600	Tank	1980	Operating
	BN-800	Russia	2,100	800	Tank	(2009)	Under construction

This table was specially prepared by the Japan Nuclear Cycle Development Institute in 2003.
[1] Achieved as the Mark-1 (MK-1) core. Modification to MK-2 core (100 MWt) was started in 1982 to improve irradiation capability.
First criticality of the MK-2 core was achieved in the same year. Present core is the MK-3 (140 MWt). Initial criticality was completed in July 2003 and now is undergoing systems testing.
[2] Reactor vessel of the loop type FBR is smaller, hence easier to make earthquake resistant compared with the tank type FBR.
In the tank type FBR, however, both the primary cooling system and IHX are contained in the reactor vessel, so the entire system is more compact.

Table A.13 Current status of final disposal programs of high-level radioactive waste in the world (2003)

Country	Selection of final disposal sites	Disposal facility	Waste type	Start of operation
Finland	Olkiluoto, Eurajoki (final disposal site)	Depth: 500 m Area: 0.15 km^2 Length of repository tunnels: 13 km	Spent fuel (BWR, VVER)	2020
USA	Yucca Mountain, Nevada (final disposal site)	Depth: 200–500 m Area: 4.65 km^2 Length of repository tunnels: 56 km	Spent fuel (BWR, PWR, etc.) Vitrified waste (mainly from national defense work)	2010
Sweden	1) Oskarshamn 2) Osthammar (candidate sites)	Depth: 400–700 m Area: 1–2 km^2 Length of repository tunnels: 45 km	Spent fuel (BWR, PWR)	~2007 2015 (Initial operation) 2023 (Regular operation)
Germany	Gorleben, Niedersachsen (site selection under reconsideration)	Depth: 840–1,200 m Area: undecided	Vitrified waste and spent fuel (PWR, BWR, etc.)	~2030
France	Undecided	Depth: unfixed Area: unfixed	Vitrified waste and spent fuel (PWR, etc.)	Undecided
Switzerland	Undecided	Depth: 400–1,000 m Area: unfixed	Vitrified waste and spent fuel (BWR, PWR)	2050
Japan	Undecided (under public solicitation for selection of the site since 2002)	Depth: more than 300 m Area: unfixed	Vitrified waste (BWR, PWR, etc.)	~2040

This table was specially prepared by the Japan Nuclear Cycle Development Institute in 2003.

Index